Wild, Food and Fitness

REVITALIZING MODERN HEALTH WITH ANCESTRAL WISDOM

REMY VISHWAKARMA

Copyright © 2012 Author Name

All rights reserved.

ISBN: 9798864183274

DEDICATION

To my all Mentors…

CONTENTS

Wild, Food and Fitness

ACKNOWLEDGMENTS

The journey of creating "Wild, Food, and Fitness: Revitalizing Modern Health with Ancestral Wisdom" has been a labor of love and collaboration, and there are many individuals and sources of inspiration we wish to acknowledge.

To our co-authors, whose expertise and passion have infused each chapter with depth and insight, we extend our deepest gratitude. Your dedication to this project has been unwavering, and your contributions have enriched this book immeasurably.

To the experts and researchers whose work has shaped the content of this book, thank you for your dedication to advancing our understanding of nutrition, fitness, and holistic wellbeing.

To the individuals who generously shared their personal stories and experiences, your contributions have added a layer of authenticity and relatability to our exploration of ancestral wisdom.

To our families and friends, who provided support, encouragement, and understanding during the long hours of research and writing, we are grateful for your unwavering belief in our mission.

To our readers, who embark on this journey of discovery with us, thank you for your curiosity, open-mindedness, and commitment to improving your own health and wellbeing.

And finally, to the ancient cultures and traditions that have shared their wisdom with the world, we honor your legacy and are humbled by the timeless knowledge you have bequeathed to us.

This book is a testament to the power of collective wisdom, and it is our hope that it serves as a source of inspiration and transformation for all who engage with its pages.

With gratitude and appreciation,

Remy Vishwakarma
Co-founder, KFS

FORWARD

Nourishing Body and Soul

In the modern era, where screens and schedules often dominate our lives, it's easy to forget the profound connection that exists between our lifestyles, our nourishment, and our physical and mental wellbeing. Yet, buried deep within our collective memory, there is a timeless wisdom that whispers to us—a wisdom that is rooted in the ancient ways of our ancestors.

"Wild, Food, and Fitness: Revitalizing Modern Health with Ancestral Wisdom" is a remarkable journey into the heart of this wisdom. It is a profound exploration of how our ancestors, the primal custodians of Earth, lived in harmony with the natural world, and how their lifestyle choices were intrinsically tied to their physical fitness and mental clarity.

In this captivating book, you will embark on a voyage through time, guided by an author who is not just a masterful storyteller but a passionate advocate for reclaiming our primal connection. You will discover how the primal blueprint of our ancestors can serve as a compass in our modern world, helping us navigate the bewildering landscape of fad diets, sedentary routines, and the disconnection from the natural world that has become all too common.

As you delve into the chapters that follow, you'll unearth a treasure trove of insights. You'll explore the vibrant tapestry of global food cultures, dive into the depths of ancient culinary traditions, and uncover the secrets of optimal nutrition and physical fitness. You'll be inspired by the stories of ancient civilizations, the resilience of indigenous cultures, and the transformative power of embracing a more primal way of life.

"Wild, Food, and Fitness" is not just a book; it's a guide, a mentor, and a source of inspiration. It offers a roadmap for those seeking to rekindle their vitality, shed the shackles of modern malaise, and rediscover the primal essence within. It is an invitation to embark on a journey of self-discovery, transformation, and wellbeing.

In a world that often feels chaotic and disconnected, this book serves as a reminder that the wisdom of our ancestors still echoes in our hearts. It invites us to return to our roots, to nurture our bodies and souls with the wisdom of the ages, and to forge a path towards lasting health and happiness.

So, as you turn the pages of "Wild, Food, and Fitness," let this be more than just a book; let it be your guide back to the primal rhythms of life, your companion on a journey of self-rediscovery, and your key to unlocking the secrets of holistic health and fitness.

May your reading journey be as enriching and transformative as the wisdom it imparts.

With heartfelt anticipation,

Remy Vishwakarma

INTRODUCTION

The Primal Connection - Lifestyle and Fitness

In the vast annals of human history, there exists a time when our ancestors lived in harmony with nature, subsisting on the bounty of the earth, and moving with the primal rhythms of life. These ancient people, often referred to as "primitive," lived a lifestyle starkly different from our modern, sedentary existence. They were the ultimate survivors, sculpted by evolution to adapt, endure, and thrive in a world filled with challenges and uncertainties.

The relationship between the lifestyle of these primal people and their fitness was not a mere coincidence; it was a fundamental aspect of their existence. In this introductory chapter, we embark on a journey to explore the profound connection between the primal way of life and physical fitness. We'll delve into the ways in which our ancestors' daily activities, dietary habits, and close bond with nature not only ensured their survival but also honed their bodies into finely tuned instruments of strength, agility, and endurance.

The Primal Blueprint

Imagine a life where every action, from hunting for food to seeking shelter, demanded physical effort and skill. Our primal ancestors were engaged in a constant dance with their environment. They climbed trees, foraged for edible plants, and navigated treacherous terrains. They were hunters, gatherers, and nomads, always on the move. These activities were not just chores but opportunities for physical exertion and development.

Physical Fitness as a Survival Imperative

In this primal existence, physical fitness was not a luxury but a necessity. The ability to sprint after prey, haul heavy loads, and scale obstacles meant the difference between survival and peril. Over time, the human body adapted to these demands, becoming a remarkably versatile and robust machine.

Dietary Wisdom of Primal Nutrition

Our ancestors' diet was equally elemental. They consumed whole foods, unaltered by the processes of modern agriculture and industry. Their plates were adorned with lean meats, foraged fruits and vegetables, nuts, seeds, and the occasional feast following a successful hunt. Their diet provided the essential nutrients required for survival and, importantly, physical vitality.

The Modern Divergence

In today's world, our lifestyles have diverged drastically from our primal roots. We've traded our spears and bows for office chairs and smartphones, and our meals have transformed into processed, convenience-driven creations. This shift in lifestyle and diet has led to a host of modern maladies, from obesity to chronic diseases, as we grapple with the consequences of our increasingly sedentary and disconnected lives.

Rediscovering the Primal Connection

However, the primal connection to fitness and wellbeing is not lost to history. In recent times, there has been a resurgence of interest in returning to a more natural way of living and eating. The paleo movement, for instance, seeks to embrace aspects of our ancestral lifestyle to promote better health and fitness.

This book, "Wild, Food, and Fitness: Revitalizing Modern Health with Ancestral Wisdom," will take you on a comprehensive journey through the wisdom of our primal ancestors. We'll explore how their lifestyle, dietary choices, and deep connection with nature are not just relics of the past but timeless lessons that can help us rekindle our own fitness, vitality, and wellbeing.

SECTION I

Back to Our Roots: Unearthing Ancestral Eating The Primal Connection - Lifestyle and Fitness

1
THE DAWN OF CULINARY AWARENESS

Imagine, if you will, a world untouched by the bustle of modern life—a landscape where the very pulse of the Earth can be felt underfoot, and where the rhythm of nature dictates the unfolding of each day. Let's step back, way back, to a time where our ancestors stood on the sprawling expanses of untamed lands, gazing upon the boundless possibilities that lay before them. It was here, in this rugged wilderness, that the embers of culinary awareness were first kindled, casting a gentle, warming light upon the raw canvas of humanity's dietary journey.

In the primal world, every rustle in the underbrush and whisper of the wind told a story—a story of survival, of opportunities, of dangers, and, most vitally, of sustenance. Our ancient forebears, with keen senses honed by the unforgiving yet bountiful natural world, forged their path, guided by an intrinsic understanding of the flora and fauna that surrounded them.

Picture yourself there, amidst the sprawling wilds, where the fruits of the land and sea lay, waiting to be discovered, understood, and, eventually, consumed. Every root unearthed, every fruit tasted, and every creature encountered, opened new chapters in the primal culinary narrative, providing not only nourishment but also vital lessons that would cascade through generations.

In the crucible of survival, a keen awareness blossomed within these early humans—an awareness of the delicate balance between nourishment and necessity. A fallen fruit, a beehive perched high above, or a herd of mammoth ambling in the distance, each presented not just a meal, but a mosaic of flavors, textures, and vital energies to be deciphered and revered.

Their palate, untainted by the synthesized flavors we know today, could discern the subtle, earthy sweetness of a freshly unearthed tuber or the rich, robust umami of sun-dried meat. They learned, through a symphony of successes and missteps, which berries tantalized the taste buds and which spelled disaster; which plants eased pain and which ones invoked it.

The introduction of fire, oh, that transformative flame, reshaped not just the foods they ate but the very fabric of their societal and nutritional evolution. Fire not only tamed the wildness of meats and plants but also unshackled a spectrum of flavors and textures previously unknown. It offered safety from pathogens, unlocked new nutrient potentials, and created opportunities for shared moments around the warmth of communal hearths.

Can you smell the intoxicating aroma of meat gently caramelizing over an open flame? Can you hear the sizzling and crackling as juices kiss the embers below? These moments around the fire were not merely instances of nutritional intake; they were sacred junctures where stories, experiences, and wisdom were shared, forging bonds that went beyond mere survival.

As we embark together on this exploration through the tapestry of ancestral eating, let's carry with us the curiosity and reverence that our ancestors held towards the natural world. We'll unearth the wisdom embedded in ancient soils, rediscovering the intrinsic connection between the earth, our food, and our inherent vitality.

With each step back in time, let's allow the ancient whispers of our forebears to guide our understanding of what it means to nourish not only our bodies but our collective spirit. For it was through their trials, triumphs, discoveries, and innovations that the seeds of culinary awareness were sown, blossoming into the rich, diverse, and complex relationship with food that continues to nourish and inspire us today.

2

THE HUNTER-GATHERER'S DIET

Here we stand, in the echoing halls of history, peering into the lives of our forebears with a kindred curiosity that ties us to them, albeit separated by the sands of time. In our last encounter, we traversed through the dawn of culinary awareness, sensing the crackling fires and tasting the initial sparks of discovery. Now, let's saunter further down this ancient path and immerse ourselves in the world of the hunter-gatherers.

Imagine being enveloped by the boundless embrace of nature, where your survival hinges upon the keenness of your senses, the prowess of your skills, and an intimate knowledge of the land's ebbs and flows. Welcome to the life of a hunter-gatherer, where each day is a new chapter of adventure, challenge, and unwavering reliance on the bounty of Mother Earth.

Our ancestors, with eyes agleam with both wariness and wonder, traversed through dense forests, open savannas, and along bounteous coastlines, foraging and hunting, sustaining themselves with the natural provisions scattered across these diverse landscapes. Picture yourself amidst a patch of berries, gleaming like jewels under the sun's gentle caress. A straightforward snack? Not quite. Each pluck, each taste was a lesson, a story – some sweet and safe, others a dangerous dalliance with the perilous games of trial and error.

Now, venture with me to the heart-pounding thrill of the hunt – the intense focus, the surge of adrenaline, and the intricate dance of predator and prey. The pursuit of game was more than a mere chase; it was a deeply spiritual journey that demanded respect for the life taken to sustain another. This was not hunting for sport, but a sacred transaction, threaded with gratitude and survival.

And oh, the vast menu they curated! From the robust, nutrient-dense meats of megafauna to the multitude of plant species – each morsel held a distinct place in their diet, providing not just sustenance but a kaleidoscope of flavors that danced upon their ancient palates. Consider the wild greens, roots, nuts, seeds, and fruits, each with its own season, its own time, and its own story to tell. Their diets, diverse and seasonally driven, were a colorful mosaic, dynamically adapting with the shifting tapestries of the seasons.

Imagine, if you will, the taste of freshly foraged mushrooms, earthy and umami, or the succulent sweetness of a ripe, sun-kissed berry, freshly plucked and still warm from the protective embrace of nature. Visualize sharing a meal, cooked over an open flame, with your tribe, under a blanket of stars, exchanging tales of the day's exploits, and reveling in the shared triumphs and tribulations of a life lived close to the earth.

In the world of the hunter-gatherer, every element of the environment, every creature, and every plant held significance. They recognized the intrinsic balance of nature, understanding that taking necessitated giving, and that respecting the cycles and inhabitants of the natural world was paramount for harmonious existence.

Our journey through the gastronomic tapestry of the hunter-gatherers paves the way for deeper insights into how these ancient practices have shaped our relationship with food and the natural world today. As we continue our exploration, may we hold in our hearts the essence of reverence, sustainability, and community that guided our ancestors, allowing it to infuse our modern perspectives and practices with a renewed sense of connection and respect.

3

TOOLS AND TECHNIQUES OF PRIMITIVE COOKING

In our last chapter, we trekked alongside our hunter-gatherer ancestors, savoring the wild bounty that nourished their daily lives. Today, let's linger a while and explore something utterly fascinating: the primitive tools and techniques that amplified the culinary experiences of our forebears. Shall we?

Now, imagine the hands of an ancestor, toughened by the wild yet capable of crafting with incredible ingenuity and finesse. With nothing but the raw materials provided by nature, they sculpted a culinary world rich in flavors, textures, and aromas, armed with an array of rudimentary yet remarkably effective tools and techniques.

Picture the first primitive tools: stones cracked and shaped into early knives, the hollowed bones that became rudimentary utensils, and the animal hides that served as containers for carrying and storing precious liquids and foods. Their hands, wielding these ancient implements, became the first chefs' hands, manipulating fire, water, earth, and air to transform raw ingredients into something truly transcendent.

The sizzle of meat as it hits the hot rocks beside a fire, can you hear it? The scent wafting upwards, infusing the air with a tantalizing aroma that speaks to something deeply primal within us. This was not mere sustenance; this was an experience, an art born from the necessity and the instinctual human drive to create and savor.

Fire, that transformative element, became the fulcrum upon which the culinary world pivoted. It wasn't merely about tossing a slab of meat into the flames. Oh no, our ancestors discovered the art of controlling heat, using slow-burning embers for gentle cooking or robust flames for searing and quick preparations.

Consider the artful technique of pit roasting – a deer, carefully prepared, swaddled in leaves, and buried with hot stones, slowly transforming underground into a tender, flavorful feast, ready to provide sustenance to the tribe above. Or imagine the slow simmering of gathered roots and herbs in a hide pouch, gradually extracting flavors and nutrients, creating a nourishing broth that would warm and sustain them through a chilly night.

And let's not forget the miracle of preservation! Drying, smoking, fermenting – these age-old techniques allowed our ancestors to harness the seasons, to capture the abundance of more plentiful times and carry them like cherished memories into the leaner months. The first dried fruits, jerked meats, and fermented concoctions were not just survival foods but flavor adventures that bridged the gap between scarcity and abundance.

The vessels, too, forged from clay or hewn from wood and stone, weren't mere containers but culinary canvases, allowing foods to be boiled, steamed, and stored. Picture a pot, crafted from the very earth upon which they stood, cradling a stew that bubbled and danced over the flickering flames.

These primitive tools and techniques paved the way for culinary innovations that span across millennia. With each cracked stone, each simmering pot, and each smoke-infused morsel, our ancestors laid the foundations upon which our diverse global cuisines now stand.

As we continue to meander through the rich landscapes of our shared culinary history, may we carry with us a newfound appreciation for the ancient hands that shaped, crafted, and created. In their resourcefulness and creativity, we find the echoes of our own culinary curiosities, bridging the past to our present in each shared meal, each story told, and each flavor savored.

4
FORAGING: NATURE'S ABUNDANT PANTRY

Welcome back, intrepid traveler, to the vibrant tapestry of our ancestral culinary adventure! Let's turn the page from primitive cooking tools and techniques to embrace a new chapter together. Today, immerse yourself in the lush, rich, and boundless pantry of the wild as we delve into the art and essence of foraging.

Picture this: a vast, untamed wilderness stretching endlessly in every direction, each leaf, berry, and root holding the whisper of nourishment and the spirit of the earth. This was the supermarket of our ancestors, a sprawling, uncontained repository of flavors, textures, and vital sustenance. Through every meander in the dense woods and every trek across open fields, a plethora of edible wonders awaited discovery and appreciation.

As the first light of day kisses the land, imagine wandering through this lush, vibrant world with a basket woven from grasses and reeds. Your senses are in a perpetual dance, discerning between the subtle, sweet fragrance of an edible berry and the slightly askew scent of its toxic look-alike. Your fingers gently caress the leaves and stems, guided by the wisdom passed through generations about which plants bless with nourishment and which ones curse with malady.

Underneath the robust trees, a carpet of mushrooms reveals itself, some offering a hearty meal and others, a dangerous game of roulette. Each step, every choice, is guided by a symbiotic relationship with the land, a deep understanding that must always respect, honor, and give back to the generous earth.

Consider the roots, concealed beneath the soil, each one a treasure chest of nutrients and flavors waiting to be unearthed. The rich, earthy scent of freshly dug tubers speaks of hearty meals around the fire, where stories and sustenance are shared in equal measure.

Up above, the boughs of trees are laden with fruits, each one a sweet, succulent reward for the keen-eyed and nimble-fingered forager. The first bite into a sun-warmed fruit, juices trickling down your chin, is a sweet symphony, a moment of pure, unadulterated connection with the world from which we sprang.

The art of foraging isn't merely about taking. It's a delicate dialogue between human and habitat, an ongoing exchange that requires giving thanks, understanding sustainability, and ensuring the bounties of today also bless the generations of tomorrow. To forage is to step into a covenant with the earth, to vow to protect, respect, and cherish every root taken, every berry plucked.

As you delve into the intricacies and anecdotes of foraging in this chapter, may you find a renewed appreciation for every morsel that graces your plate today. Envision the lush, wild pantry of our ancestors, and reflect upon the remarkable journey of humanity from those ancient, echoing forests and fields to the vast array of foods that grace our modern tables.

In "Wild, Food, and Fitness," we intertwine the ancient wisdom of our ancestors with our contemporary quest for health and wellbeing. Let the stories, the practices, and the ancient symbiosis with nature guide your steps as you navigate through your own journey of food, fitness, and a deeply rooted connection with the world around us.

5

SEAFOOD AND THE ANCIENT MARINER DIET

Together, let's set our sails and embark upon a maritime journey, exploring how the ocean's treasure trove of seafood enriched and diversified the diet of our forebears.

Close your eyes for a moment, and imagine standing on a primordial shoreline. The sea, vast and infinite, kisses the land with frothy waves, whispering tales of distant shores and underwater realms abundant with life. Our ancestors, with eyes gleaming with reflection of azure depths, witnessed the sea not just as a formidable expanse to be conquered, but as a generous provider, teeming with nourishment.

Seafood was more than mere sustenance for the ancient mariner; it was a world of flavors to be explored and cherished. Picture the deft hands of an experienced fisher, casting handmade nets into the shimmering waters, awaiting the telltale tug of a bounteous catch. Or imagine the skilled spear-fisher, merging with the undulating underwater world, anticipating the darting movement of a succulent fish.

Oysters, crabs, fish, mussels... the ocean bestowed upon them a banquet, ever-changing with the tides and seasons. Each catch was a gift, to be respected and utilized to its fullest. The fresh, saline scent of the ocean mingled with the earthy aroma of seaweed and the tantalizing smokiness of a nearby fire, where today's catch sizzled, destined to nourish and delight.

The diverse palette of flavors from the sea — sweet shellfish, umami-rich seaweed, and the delicate flesh of fish — became interwoven with the mariners' very being. Each meal was a celebration of the sea's generosity and a testament to the skills and knowledge of those who harvested its riches.

But the mariner diet wasn't just a hedonistic indulgence of flavors. With every bite, vital nutrients from the sea's bounty — omega-3 fatty acids, iodine, zinc, and a host of vitamins — coursed through their veins, fueling their expeditions and ensuring survival amidst the challenges of maritime life.

Consider, too, the ingenuity of preservation at sea: the salting, drying, and fermenting of seafood that allowed these nourishing foods to be stored and enjoyed far from the ocean's embrace. In every preserved fish or seaweed, there existed not just a safeguard against scarcity but a tangible, flavorful connection to the memories of bountiful harvests and shared meals beside the lapping waves.

As we delve into the stories, techniques, and flavors of the ancient mariner diet, perhaps we may find an echo of their respect for the ocean and its creatures in our own seafood practices today. Let's honor the age-old bond between humanity and the sea, navigating through the annals of history with an appreciation for the maritime cultures and their ageless, salt-kissed wisdom.

6 CEREALS, GRAINS, AND EARLY AGRICULTURE

In this chapter, we will tread lightly through the birthplace of agriculture, gleaning whispers from the fields that witnessed the germination of both seed and civilization: the world of cereals and grains.

Picture it: the vast expanse of wild, waving grasses, each blade nursing precious kernels, an embodiment of life's perpetuating dance. The first people who discovered the secret within these seeds could not have fathomed the revolution they would sow, intertwining our destinies with these humble grains forever.

The tale of grains is as rich and varied as the soils that have cradled them throughout millennia. Our ancestors, once bound to the whims of wild bounty, found in grains the miraculous potential to root their tribes, to foster communities that would stand resilient against the flow of seasons and the migration of herds.

The hand that first sowed wild wheat, barley, and millet into the nurturing earth wove a new chapter in our collective story, a chapter that entwined the fates of human and grain in a symbiotic dance of growth, harvest, and renewal.

The scent of the first milled flour and the warmth from the inaugural loaves of freshly baked bread... can you sense it? These primal loaves, rough and hearty, became symbols of shared prosperity, of the security afforded by a stored harvest, and of the generosity of the earth that cradled each seedling.

Delve deeper and envision the sprawling fields cultivated by the early farmers, each furrow an embodiment of hope and anticipation. The turning of the seasons brought the whispering winds through stalks of ripened grains, each rustle singing praises of abundance and life.

But our ancestors knew that with this bounty came new responsibilities and challenges. The need to guard their fields, to understand the whims of weather and soil, and to store their harvest away from pest and decay - agriculture bound them to new labors even as it sowed seeds of stability and community.

Cereals and grains, however, were not merely staples of sustenance. They became venerated symbols of life, death, and rebirth - spiritual icons rooted deeply within the culture and beliefs of the people. In every seed, there existed a promise of tomorrow, a tangible whisper of the divine, a pulsating heartbeat of the community.

And yet, with every bite of bread or sip of early grain-based brew, we are reminded that the stories of grains are not simply tales of life and nourishment but are intertwined with the ancient cultural tapestries that echo through our modern culinary and agricultural landscapes.

Dear reader, as we wander through the golden fields of early agriculture in "Wild, Food, and Fitness," may you find seeds of wisdom and inspiration from our forebears who tread softly upon the fertile earth. Let the tales of their toils, discoveries, and innovations germinate within, nurturing your own journey through the rich, expansive plains of nutrition, health, and ancestral wisdom.

7
THE DOMESTICATION OF LIVESTOCK

As we nestle into this exploration, allow me to guide you through verdant pastures and ancient homesteads, where we'll discover the profound and transformative practice that forever shaped our relationship with the animal kingdom: the domestication of livestock.

Envision, for a moment, vast landscapes where wild creatures roam, each animal a living embodiment of the wild, untamed nature that cradled our ancestors. And there, amidst the wild, a profound connection took root, intertwining the destinies of humans and beasts in a symbiotic dance that would echo through the eons.

In the gentle bleat of a sheep, the bellow of a cow, and the cluck of a hen, our forebears heard the harmonies of sustenance, kinship, and mutual survival. As they began to tenderly coax these creatures from the wild into the nascent semblance of domesticity, they unknowingly sculpted the architecture of civilizations yet to come.

The stories woven into the domestication of livestock are as diverse and varied as the tapestry of cultures that dot our global heritage. Every creature that stepped from the wild into the human fold brought with it not merely sustenance in the form of meat, milk, and eggs, but also an opportunity to plow fields, to craft garments, and to traverse distant lands.

Imagine the first tender moments shared between human and beast – a gently extended hand offering nourishment, an initial bond forged in the crucible of trust and necessity. This was a relationship, after all, that transcended mere survival, unfolding into a rich narrative that cherished the animal not merely as a provider but as a sacred, vital being within the community.

The narrative of domestication is also one of reverence and responsibility. As our ancestors welcomed these beings into their lives, they embraced the duty to provide, protect, and honor every life that sustained their own. Animals were celebrated in myth, revered in ritual, and respected in death.

We'll explore, together, how the domestication of livestock nurtured not just the physical bodies of our ancestors but also their spiritual and cultural lives. Through every drop of milk and each woven strand of wool, the animals became irrevocably interwoven into the cultural, spiritual, and everyday lives of the people.

The paths we'll tread in this chapter will guide us through the myriad ways in which livestock shaped our culinary and cultural landscapes. As we explore, let us reflect upon the sacredness of the bonds forged between ancient herders and their charges, and ponder how these relationships can guide our modern engagements with the creatures that continue to sustain and enrich our lives.

Imagine, the first symbiotic moments when human hands nurtured animal kin with offerings of food and shelter, and in return, the animals, with their unspoken gratitude, enriched human lives with sustenance and vitality.

The Bovine Sustenance

Cows, with their calm, languid eyes, entered the human narrative not merely as providers of rich, nourishing milk and hearty meat but also as beings of gentle strength, capable of tilling the fields to usher forth a bounty of crops. Ponder upon the serene pastures where cattle grazed under the watchful eyes of their human caretakers. Within these interactions, a foundational understanding was formed, recognizing that nurturing the wellbeing of these bovine companions directly correlated to the prosperity and nourishment of the human community.

Shepherding through Generations

Now, wander alongside the ancient shepherds, who, under the vast expanse of starlit skies, safeguarded their woolly charges from predators and perils. Sheep offered not just succulent morsels and warm wool but also became woven into the stories and songs that echoed across the rolling hills and through time. Every sheepfold told tales of legacy and lineage, where knowledge, tales, and shepherding skills were inherited through the whisperings from one generation to the next.

In the Company of Swine

Venture forth into the forests and fields where early farmers discovered the symbiotic potential of pigs - creatures capable of transforming scraps and forage into delectable nourishment. Picture the diversity of breeds, each uniquely adapted to the landscapes they inhabited and the communities they nurtured. The pig, through its own vitality and resourcefulness, augmented the lives of our forebears, contributing to a robust, varied diet, and enlivening feasts and celebrations.

Poultry and the Gift of Eggs

Imagine the harmonious clucking of hens in ancient homesteads, where eggs, a symbol of life and fertility, were revered and cherished as a daily bounty. Chickens, with their spirited energy and diligent scratching and pecking, not only provided sustenance but also kept the pest populations in check, safeguarding the grains and crops that sustained the community.

The Cultural Mosaic

Our journey would be incomplete without recognizing how the domestication of livestock painted vibrant strokes upon the cultural canvas. Animals, through their beings and the products they provided, were interwoven into the spiritual, mythical, and practical tapestries of daily life. They became symbols of deity, prosperity, and survival, enriching the cultural expressions through art, mythology, and societal structures.

A Covenant of Respect

As we wander through these ancient landscapes, let's also reflect upon the sacred covenant forged between human and animal. With every life taken, an unspoken promise was honored – to respect, to thank, and to remember. Rituals and ceremonies blossomed from this sacred bond, ensuring that the animals who gave their lives were honored through mindful utilization of every part, and through the stories and gratitude passed down through epochs.

8

FERMENTATION: PRESERVING AND FLAVORING

Today, let us delve into a fascinating chapter, where the magic of microbiology intertwines with the culinary arts, creating a melody of flavors and safeguarding nourishment through time: welcome to the world of fermentation.

Imagine, if you will, a time where refrigeration was a distant future concept and where the preservation of food was not just a need but an art form enveloped in mystery and wonder. Our ancestors, through observation, intuition, and perhaps a dash of serendipity, discovered a method to safeguard their precious harvests and enhance their culinary experiences: they unlocked the secrets of fermentation.

The Magic of Microbes

Dive with me into the microcosm of the fermenting vessel, where invisible beings – yeasts, bacteria, and fungi – toil diligently, transforming grains, fruits, vegetables, and milk into tantalizing symphonies of flavor and fortitude. The ancient people did not merely find a way to preserve their sustenance but, in the microcosmic dance of fermentation, discovered new, exciting dimensions of taste, texture, and aroma.

A Vessel of Vitality

Embark on a journey through time and culture, exploring how different civilizations crafted their unique fermented signatures: from the robust, complex flavors of kimchi in Korea to the effervescent vivacity of kombucha in China, and the hearty, soulful depths of sauerkraut in Europe. Each ferment, in its unique way, became a vessel that cradled the vitality and culinary identity of the cultures from whence they emerged.

Grains and Goblets

Now, wander through golden fields of barley and rice, where the grains were not only destined to become sustenance for the body but also libations for the soul. Sip, in your imagination, on the ancient beers and sake, where every drop held the essence of the earth and the toil of those who nurtured it, bridging communities together in shared celebration, reverence, and camaraderie.

Cheese: A Tapestry of Terroir

Journey through the rolling pastures and into the cheese caves, where milk, with the gentle coaxing of microbes and time, transformed into myriad forms of cheese. Each wheel, a tapestry of the land, the animals, and the hands that crafted it, matured into a rich mosaic of flavors, textures, and aromas, weaving a story that transcended time and space.

The Healing Brine

Let's explore the potent world of pickling, where vegetables submerged in a brine were reborn into zesty, lively, and nourishing morsels. Not merely a method of preservation, the pickling crock also emerged as a crucible where medicinal herbs and spices mingled with the vegetables, creating concoctions that nurtured wellness and vitality.

Harmonizing Culinary Landscapes

In the waltz of fermentation, our ancestors found a means to harmonize with the natural world, to respectfully harness the invisible world of microbes in a symphony of preservation and culinary innovation. Through the subtle art of fermentation, they crafted bridges that connected seasons, ensuring the summer's bounty nourished them through winter's chill.

As we close this chapter, my dear reader, may the ancient alchemy of fermentation inspire you to explore, to respect, and to savor the rich, boundless landscapes of our culinary heritage. In the bubbling crock and the aging cheese, may you find echoes of our ancestors who, with intuition and respect, danced harmoniously with the microscopic world, crafting legacies of flavor, preservation, and vitality that continue to nourish and enchant our palates today. May the tales of ancient ferments guide us towards a future that respects, honors, and joyfully engages with the natural world in all its microcosmic splendor.

9

ANCIENT COOKING METHODS AND IMPLEMENTS

Let's embark together on another enchanting journey, this time immersing ourselves into the warmth of ancestral hearths to explore the age-old artistry of ancient cooking methods and implements.

Hearth and Home

Close your eyes and visualize the first hearths, where flames danced and crackled, providing warmth, light, and a focal point where communities gathered. In these sacred spaces, the art of cooking evolved from the mere act of heating food to an intricate dance of flavors and techniques, seeping deeply into the cultural identity of each tribe and civilization.

Stone, Fire, and Flavor

Journey with me to the primal landscapes where stones, heated by the robust flames of open fires, became the first griddles upon which meals were crafted. Here, our forebears skillfully grilled meats, fish, and perhaps even foraged vegetables, unlocking new dimensions of flavor, aroma, and sustenance. The mastery of fire and stone in cooking became not merely a survival strategy but an art form that would echo through millennia.

Earthenware and Culinary Alchemy

Let's traverse together to the realms where clay was shaped and fired into vessels of various forms – pots, pans, and urns that would hold the hearty stews, soups, and brews. These earthenware implements, both humble and crucial, witnessed the amalgamation of ingredients, where the melding of flavors, textures, and aromas unfolded into a myriad of delightful culinary experiences.

The Art of Smoking

Venture into the woody groves where our ancestors discovered the magic of smoking – an age-old technique to preserve and embolden the flavors of meat, fish, and perhaps even cheese and vegetables. The smoke, infused with the spirit of the wood, delicately caressed and permeated the fibers of the food, imparting a depth of flavor and preservation that enabled sustenance to be enjoyed across seasons.

Underground Ovens and Earth's Embrace

Now, let us dig deep into the earth, exploring the subterranean ovens where food was gently enveloped in the warm embrace of Mother Earth. The underground cooking methods, witnessed in various cultures across the globe, bestowed upon the ingredients the slow, nurturing heat that tenderized, caramelized, and harmoniously melded every element into a unified, sumptuous whole.

The Beauty of Baking

We shall wander into the aromatic domain of ancient ovens, where dough – simple yet profound – was transformed through the gentle caress of heat into hearty, soul-nourishing bread. The freshly baked loaves, embodying the essence of grains and the whisper of yeast, emerged as symbols of sustenance, community, and the benevolent abundance of the earth.

Spits and Grills: A Dance of Flames

And lastly, let's explore the world of spits and grills, where food was kissed by open flames, creating a delicate char and an enticing, primal flavor that has transcended time and culture. Here, amidst the flickering light and the seductive aromas, ancient chefs masterfully balanced the elements of heat and timing to perfect the art of grilling.

The Pots that Shaped Civilization

As we further simmer into our exploration, let's delve into the unassuming yet revolutionary world of pottery. Each vessel, molded from the humble earth, tells a story of the people who shaped it, painting a portrait of their daily lives, diets, and culinary traditions. Whether perched over open flames or nestled amid ash, these pots silently bore witness to the slow-bubbling stews and broths, embodying the patience and nurturing care of the hands that crafted them.

The Primitive Oven's Evolution

Envision, if you will, the evolution of the primitive oven, gradually refining through the epochs from mere fire pits to enclosed spaces, capable of sustaining and regulating heat. The earth ovens of Polynesia, the tandoors of India, and the clay ovens of ancient Rome – each was meticulously engineered, becoming monumental in shaping regional cuisines. Through the gentle cradle of persistent heat, grains transformed into bread, meats into savory indulgences, and vegetables into mellow, sweetened delights.

The Cultural Significance of Cooking Implements

Contemplate the myriad of implements: mortars and pestles grinding grains and spices, stone slabs and planks on which dough was flattened and baked, and the various intricately constructed tools for grinding, pressing, and straining. Each implement was not merely a tool; it was a key that unlocked new possibilities in the culinary arts, enabling our ancestors to explore new textures, flavors, and combinations, and thus enhancing their quality of life.

The Gathering and the Feast

Now, allow your senses to wander through the grandeur of ancient feasts. The intricate artistry of cooking methods was not merely about sustenance but also an elaborate tapestry of community, celebration, and unity. The spits bearing sumptuous roasts, the bubbling pots of rich, hearty stews, and the ovens birthing golden, crusty bread – all of these painted a vibrant picture of abundance, shared amongst kin and kin alike.

Creating with Constraints

Explore the ingenuity birthed from constraint, as our ancestors, bound by the limitations of their environments, materials, and understanding, conjured wondrous culinary innovations. The scarcity of fuel birthed the haybox – an ancient slow cooker that utilized insulation to conserve heat and slow cook meals to perfection. Similarly, the discovery and mastery over embers allowed for slow roasting and the gradual caramelization of foods, bringing forth decadent flavors and textures.

Ancient Sweets and Confectioneries

Let's also visit the realms where sweet delights were conjured. The bakers and sweet-makers of yore, utilizing honey, fruits, and later, sugar, combined with the gentle heat of embers and ovens, crafted treats that transcended mere nourishment, becoming symbols of celebration, prosperity, and affability.

Spiritual Symbolism in Cooking

As we gently simmer towards the chapter's close, reflect upon the sacredness infused within ancient culinary practices. The fire, the vessels, and the ingredients often transcended the physical, symbolizing spiritual beliefs, celestial beings, and eternal cycles. The baking of bread, the fermenting of beverages, and the simmering of stews were deeply entwined with rituals, offerings, and ceremonies that harmonized the physical and spiritual worlds.

A Pot of Multifaceted Culinary Culture

As we continue our exploration, let's consider the multifaceted world of pottery and its impact on diverse culinary landscapes. Take, for example, the "Dok Jok," a traditional Thai flour mold crafted of brass or stainless steel. Its meticulous design brought forth the delicate beauty of Thai desserts, marrying sweet, floral, and nutty notes into an inviting tapestry of flavors.

Ingenious Innovations Across Civilizations

Conversing about the evolution of ovens, the Tandoor oven from the Indian subcontinent is a quintessential example of this innovation. Enveloped by a rich, cultural history, the Tandoor masterfully grills meats and bakes bread like the beloved Naan and Roti, all whilst imparting a distinct, smoky flavor – a signature of many Indian delicacies.

The Stone Grinders of Mesoamerica

Reflect upon the Mesoamerican "Metate," a stone tool used by indigenous peoples to grind corn, spices, and cocoa. The rhythmic grinding of ingredients between stone surfaces not only sculpted the flavors of the region but also shaped the culinary narrative of civilizations, fostering communal gatherings and crafting dishes that remain timeless.

Celebratory and Sustenance Cooking

In ancient Greece, the clay-plastered "Clibanus" was more than an oven – it was an implement of celebration and everyday life. From savoring the sweetness of honey-drenched Loukoumades to the hearty, nourishing flavors of lamb and vegetable stews, the Clibanus illustrated how cooking transcended sustenance, weaving into the very social and spiritual tapestry of society.

The Beauty of Limitation-Induced Innovation

Diving into the ingenious world of culinary contraptions, let's linger upon the Japanese "Kamado," an earthen stove that perfectly encapsulates innovation birthed from constraints. Utilizing charcoal as its heat source, the Kamado efficiently sustained heat, enabling the crafting of perfectly steamed rice, a staple that has cradled generations and crowned countless meals.

Sacred Culinary Rituals in Ancient Egypt

Enveloping our senses in the sacrosanct world of spiritual culinary practices, ancient Egypt's beer brewing artistry is a luminescent thread in the tapestry of culinary spirituality. Revered not just as a beverage but as an offering to the gods, the brewing and consumption of beer were intertwined with prayers, rituals, and a profound respect for the divine sustenance provided.

The Soulful Sweets of the Middle Ages

Finally, let's meander through the spice-infused world of medieval confectionery. The "Lebkuchener," a gingerbread maker, emerged not only as a craftsman but also as an artist, crafting shapes, symbols, and messages into the molasses-darkened dough. Embellished with honey, nuts, and spices, these sweets were a rich, soulful celebration of both everyday life and festive occasions.

Our journey through the antiquated world of ancient cooking methods and implements nudges us to peer through the lens of time, embracing the multifaceted culinary innovations and practices of our forebears. From the smoky Tandoors of India to the sweet, spice-laden confections of medieval Europe, every implement, technique, and creation is a thread, intricately woven into the boundless, vibrant tapestry of our shared culinary heritage.

May we savor each tale, each flavor, and each whisper of ancestral wisdom, allowing them to infuse our modern kitchens and plates with a reverence for the past, an appreciation for the present, and an anticipation for the future culinary adventures that await.

10
CULINARY TRADITIONS AND RITUALS

A Seat at the Ancestral Table

This isn't just about the ingredients or the techniques but the heart, soul, and essence behind them. Ever wondered why certain dishes are integral to festivals or why some foods are considered auspicious in certain cultures? Well, fasten your seatbelt (or should I say apron?) because we're about to embark on a flavorful journey through time and traditions.

The Soul of a Dish Lies in Its Story

Remember grandma's comforting soup or that pie recipe passed down from generations? More than just a concoction of ingredients, they were stories simmering in those pots, tales of love, hardship, celebration, and unity. The act of preparing and consuming these dishes was like time travel, connecting us to our ancestors and the tales they told.

Mooncakes and Mid-Autumn Musings

Take, for instance, the Chinese Mid-Autumn Festival. Those beautiful, intricate mooncakes aren't just delicious; they're a symbol of reunion, of family. Legend speaks of lovers separated, messages hidden in mooncakes, and celestial beings. Every bite of that sweet, dense treat is a taste of history, myth, and familial love.

The Sacred Corn of Native Americans

Traveling to the vast expanses of North America, the Native Americans revered corn, or maize, as a sacred gift from the Creator. Ceremonies like the Green Corn Festival were not just a celebration of the harvest but a deep spiritual thanksgiving, a recognition of the balance of life. Sharing dishes made from corn was more than nutrition; it was an act of spiritual communion.

Indian Pujas and Prasadam

Over in India, the rituals are vast and varied. Yet, a common thread is the offering of 'Prasadam' – sacred food. Be it the sweet 'Pongal' during the harvest festival or the rich 'Kheer' offered to the moon goddess during Karva Chauth, these dishes, infused with devotion, are believed to carry the blessings of the divine. Sharing prasadam among devotees is not just about satiating hunger but nurturing souls.

Passover and the Symbolism of Matzah

As we hop over to Jewish traditions, the Passover meal stands out. Each element on the Seder plate, especially the unleavened bread or Matzah, tells a tale. It's a poignant reminder of the Israelites' hurried escape from Egypt, symbolizing both the affliction of slavery and the joy of freedom.

A Toast to Traditions

From the Japanese tea ceremony that encapsulates Zen philosophy and aesthetics to the Ethiopian coffee ritual that binds communities, culinary rituals are sprinkled with symbolism, shared memories, and an essence that transcends borders.

In wrapping up this flavorful journey through traditions, it's awe-inspiring to realize that every dish, every ritual, is a bridge. A bridge that connects us to our roots, our ancestors, and the collective stories of humanity. So, the next time you're relishing a festive dish or partaking in a culinary ritual, pause for a moment. Savor the flavors, the stories, the love, and the legacy. Because, dear reader, in that moment, you're not just eating; you're time traveling, soul nurturing, and tradition continuing. Cheers to the tales our food tells!

11
NUTRITIONAL WISDOM OF INDIGENOUS CULTURES

Journey to the Roots of Nutritional Prowess

Today's trail takes us through the lush valleys and rugged terrains of indigenous cultures, where every fruit, root, and leaf whispers ancient tales of nutritional wisdom. Let's explore how our forebears didn't just eat to live but mastered the art of living well through mindful eating.

Where Every Bite Speaks a Thousand Words

Imagine this: You're wandering through a thick Amazonian forest with a tribe whose ancestors have called this verdant wonderland home for centuries. Every plant, every creature is not merely a part of their environment but a chapter in their grand, nutritional encyclopedia. The indigenous people have a profound understanding that what they consume isn't merely sustenance, but a delicate dance with the environment, ensuring vitality for both the land and themselves.

The Vibrant Tapestry of Native American Cuisine

Our first stop is with the Native Americans, whose profound respect for nature is embedded in their culinary practices. Consider the "Three Sisters" – corn, beans, and squash – a triumvirate that graced many indigenous tables. Not merely chosen for their deliciousness, these sisters were cultivated together because they enriched the soil and each other. This wasn't just farming; this was an elegant, symbiotic ballet of nutrition and sustainability.

African Ingenuity in Every Morsel

We then saunter through the diverse landscapes of Africa, where traditional diets spoke to the symbiosis of flavor and function. The nutrient-dense baobab fruit, often called the "Tree of Life", not only tickled the palate but also nourished the body with its bounty of vitamin C, calcium, and antioxidants. In every bite, there's a silent thank-you whispered to the sprawling baobab tree, under whose shade countless tales have been spun.

The Polynesian Palette of Wellness

Sailing toward the idyllic islands of Polynesia, we encounter a holistic approach to eating where nothing is wasted. The breadfruit, a staple that could be roasted, boiled, or turned into flour, was more than sustenance. It was a lesson in utilizing nature's gifts to their fullest, minimizing waste, and honoring the bounty of the earth.

Aboriginal Australia's Bush Tucker

And oh, the secrets that lie within the Australian bush! Indigenous Australians perfected the art of thriving in harmony with their seemingly harsh environment. With a rich and varied "bush tucker" (bush food), including the nutritious Kakadu plum, packed with immune-boosting vitamin C, and the versatile macadamia nut, they demonstrated a deep-rooted understanding that nature, when respected, reveals her abundant pantry.

Towards a Future of Nourishing Ties

These time-honored practices, dear reader, are not just historical notes but threads that weave through the fabric of present and future nutritional wisdom. From the sustainable agriculture practices of the Native Americans to the zero-waste philosophy of the Polynesians, there's a resonance in these ancient rhythms that speaks to our modern souls.

Whispers from the Andean Highlands

Let's meander through the windswept Andean highlands where the earthy potatoes, both vibrant and subdued, and hearty quinoa have nestled in the folds of the earth for generations. The Andean communities understood the peaks and valleys of nutritional balance, creating a diet that was in harmony with the ebb and flow of their challenging environment. The potato, in its countless varieties, was more than sustenance. It was a resilient emblem of their endurance and creativity in treacherous terrains, with each tuber carrying flavors and stories from the soil it sprouted from.

The Arctic's Unyielding Embrace

Journeying to the harsh yet mesmerizing Arctic, the Inuit people tell tales of survival, adaptability, and profound respect for the life around them. In a terrain seemingly barren, their diet was surprisingly rich and diversified, extracting nutrients from the sea and land alike. The Inuit not only survived but thrived, understanding the nutritional bounty the seemingly stark landscape provided. From seals which provided vitamin-rich fat, to foraged berries bursting with antioxidants, their dietary choices wove a tapestry that was harmoniously tied to the land and sea.

The Ancient Grains of Mesopotamia

Sailing through time, let's glean ancient wisdom from the bounteous plains of Mesopotamia, often hailed as the cradle of civilization. Amidst the flourishing city-states, grains like barley and emmer wheat were not merely cultivated but revered. These ancient grains, hearty and wholesome, were entwined with myths, deities, and daily life, symbolizing fertility and abundance. The

Mesopotamians, with their irrigation dexterity and granary systems, transformed these grains into a myriad of dishes that nourished civilizations and facilitated culinary and cultural exchanges.

The Mediterranean's Bounteous Shores

Floating towards the warm, embracing breezes of the Mediterranean, we uncover a tapestry where every olive, grape, and fig holds a secret to longevity and vitality. This isn't just a diet; it's a philosophy where meals are savored, where eating is a communal celebration, and where every ingredient plays a role in wellness and pleasure alike. Olives, for instance, were cherished not just for their robust, versatile flavors but for their heart-healthy fats and antioxidant properties, embodying the essence of Mediterranean living – savoring wholesomeness in every bite and moment.

The Spice-Infused Trails of India

Ah, India! A land where spices are not merely condiments but the soul of a dish, whispering tales of trade, invasions, and exploration. Turmeric, the golden-hued healer, was a staple in every kitchen, not just for its warm, earthy flavors but for its potent anti-inflammatory and antioxidant properties. Ginger, pepper, cardamom... each spice was a note in a harmonious melody, contributing not just to the symphony of flavors but to the balance and wellness of the body.

Through every terrain and time, these culinary narratives unfurl, revealing that our ancestors were not just surviving, but harmoniously coexisting with nature, understanding and unlocking its myriad secrets. Their culinary choices were inscribed with an innate wisdom that nourished their bodies, safeguarded their health, and fortified their connection with the earth.

In every grain, root, fruit, and leaf, there is knowledge waiting to be revered and passed down. As we forge forward, creating our own culinary tales, may we sip on the ancient wisdom simmering in our pots, savoring the nourishment of both body and soul, and whispering our own stories into the winds of time.

12

CASE STUDIES: EATING HABITS OF ANCIENT CIVILIZATIONS

Gathering Around the Ancient Hearth

Today we're diving deep into the archives of history, exploring the bustling marketplaces, cozy hearths, and festive feasts of yesteryears. Our quest? To unearth the dining diaries of some of the most iconic ancient civilizations.

Dining with the Pharaohs: Ancient Egypt

First stop: the golden sands of Ancient Egypt, where the Nile isn't just a river but the lifeblood nourishing the civilization. Here, in the shadows of the pyramids, bread (made from emmer wheat) was the staple, so pivotal that it even found a place in the afterlife. And oh, the beer! Not the fizzy kind we're accustomed to, but a thick, nourishing brew that was a part of daily meals. Then there were figs, dates, and lentils, creating a palette that was both simple and profound.

Feasting in the Forum: Ancient Rome

Onto the grandeur of Rome, where dining was an art, and banquets, an expression of affluence and culture. The Romans

45

cherished their olives and grapes, with wine being a central component of meals. But did you know they had a penchant for exotic flavors like garum (a fermented fish sauce) and loved their meats dressed in intricate sauces? And let's not forget the puls, a porridge made from barley, seasoned with herbs and cheese. A simple staple amidst the opulence.

Tea Tales and Rice Rituals: Ancient China

Sailing east, we land in Ancient China, where every meal is a poetic ode to balance and harmony. The Chinese, even then, mastered the art of balancing yin and yang in their meals. Rice, the cornerstone, was paired with a plethora of vegetables, meats, and sauces. And tea, more than a beverage, was an institution, a ritual symbolizing peace, reflection, and communion with nature.

The Vibrant Mayan Maize Melodies

Journeying to the mesmeric rainforests of Central America, the Mayans welcome us with their corn (or maize) celebrations. Central to their cosmology and diet, maize was revered, celebrated, and transformed into a variety of dishes, from tamales to atol (a warm maize-based drink). Accompanied by beans, chili peppers, and a rich cacao drink, the Mayan table was a colorful canvas of tastes and tales.

The Harmonious Hues of Harappan Diet

Let's tread back in time to the sophisticated city grids of the Indus Valley Civilization. Though much remains shrouded in mystery, excavations hint at a diet rich in grains, especially barley. With elaborate granaries, we can only imagine bustling markets filled with fresh produce, dairy, and perhaps even fermented drinks. The terracotta pots might have bubbled with flavorful stews, echoing the rhythms of a civilization in its prime.

The Robust Rhythms of the Viking Feast

Stepping aboard a sturdy Viking longship, we're whisked away to the smoky longhouses of Scandinavia. The Vikings, despite the icy fjords and rugged terrains, curated a diet of surprising variety and sustenance. With robust, hearty flavors derived from the ocean and the sparse vegetation, the Viking feasts were a testament to their resilience and resourcefulness. Think of dried fish, preserved in the brisk northern winds, hearty stews simmering over crackling fires, and dark, nourishing ale brewed from barley. Each bite, a tale of seafaring, exploration, and endurance against the elements.

The Exotic Enigma of the Ottoman Empire

Journeying southeast, we find ourselves amidst the bustling bazaars of the Ottoman Empire, where the air is thick with the enticing aroma of exotic spices, and the tables are laden with the produce of three continents. The Ottoman cuisine, renowned for its vivid colors and intricate flavors, was a spectacular amalgamation of Central Asian, Middle Eastern, and Balkan tastes. Pilaf, the exquisite canvas of rice, was adorned with nuts, spices, and fruits, while meats were slow-cooked to perfection, bathed in rich, nuanced sauces. The sweet finale often came in the form of baklava, a symphony of thin pastry, honey, and nuts, revealing that indulgence and sophistication have always been timeless culinary companions.

The Lush Labyrinths of Polynesia

Then let's embark upon the vibrant, lush islands of Polynesia, where the sea whispers tales of navigation, exploration, and culinary ingenuity. Taro, breadfruit, and coconuts formed the triumvirate of their diet, while the ocean bestowed its bounty in the form of fish and shellfish. The enchanting Luau feasts showcased their mastery in utilizing nature's oven – the earth, where meats and vegetables were slowly cooked to perfection, embodying the warmth and hospitality of the islands.

Gastronomic Glory of the Persian Empire

Now, imagine the sprawling Persian Empire, a land where poetry and cuisine danced in a sensual embrace. Saffron-infused rice pilafs, slowly simmered stews (Khoresh), and an array of bread like the delicate Taftoon or robust Barbari graced the tables from the bustling bazaars of Tehran to the regal courts of Persepolis. The Persians, with their sophisticated agricultural systems and storied Silk Road spices, wove a culinary tapestry that whispered tales of kings, caravans, and long-forgotten recipes.

Savoring the Simplicity of Native American Tribes

To conclude our gastronomic journey, let's explore the vast, varied terrains of North America, where diverse Native American tribes crafted diets deeply entwined with the land's spirit. From the Three Sisters (beans, corn, and squash) cultivated with profound respect for the earth, to the bison hunts on the expansive plains, their diets reflected a harmonious, sustainable relationship with nature. Stews, cornbread, and dried meats sustained tribes through seasons, migrations, and generations, embodying a wisdom that seamlessly blended sustenance with sustainability.

The echoes of ancient culinary endeavors beckon us, don't they? The myriad flavors crafted by our ancestors weren't just about sustenance but were a celebration of their environments, communities, and traditions. Each civilization, while distinct in flavor and technique, shared a universal understanding that food was not merely fuel but a sacred thread that wove through every aspect of life, binding together the physical and the spiritual, the individual and the community, the mortal and the divine.

Our culinary adventure through time invites reflection upon our modern plates: how can we weave the ancestral wisdom of sustainability, balance, and respect for our environment into our contemporary culinary practices? The answers, perhaps, simmer quietly in the pots and pans of history, waiting to be tasted and understood once more.

And so, with the echoes of ancient feasts still lingering on our palates, we'll continue our journey through time, culture, and flavor in the chapters ahead. Here's to the next delicious adventure together!

13

FOOD AND SOCIETAL STRUCTURES

Imagine we are time travelers, embarking on a journey through epochs and dynasties, exploring how societies have been shaped, often subtly yet profoundly, by something as fundamental as food. Buckle up, dear reader, for we are about to traverse through the annals of history, exploring the vibrant mosaic that depicts the profound relationship between food and societal structures.

The Cascading Influence of Crop Choices

Visualize ancient civilizations, where the choice of cultivated crops wasn't merely a dietary preference but a decision that wove the very fabric of societal interactions and structures. Rice cultivation in ancient China, for instance, required meticulously managed water systems and collective labor, fostering a society that prized community efforts and centralized governance.

Conversely, consider the wheat farmers of ancient Greece, who operated with a level of autonomy, sowing the seeds not only of hearty grains but also of a society where individuality and democratic ideas could take root and flourish.

The Emblematic Bread and Circuses

Navigate towards the Roman Empire, where "bread and circuses" wasn't merely a phrase but a calculated strategy employed by emperors to appease and control the masses. The provision of free wheat and engaging spectacles symbolized a socio-political contract where sustenance and entertainment were exchanged for political compliance and societal stability.

The Entwined Destinies of Slaves and Sugar

Our journey takes a somber turn as we encounter the deeply intertwined histories of sugar cultivation and slavery. In the vast plantations of the Caribbean and the Americas, the insatiable global demand for sugar fueled a tragically exploitative system that perpetuated societal divisions based on race and economic status. Thus, a single crop altered socio-economic structures, catalyzing wealth for some and unimaginable hardship for others.

The Caste Cuisine of India

Drifting eastwards, we explore the intricate tapestry of Indian society, where the variegated threads of caste, religion, and food practices are interwoven tightly. From the vegetarian diets of the Brahmins, symbolizing purity and piety, to the various regional and caste-specific delicacies, food became a tangible delineation of identity, social status, and cultural belonging in a multifaceted society.

The Potato's Potent Impact

Let's whisk away to Europe, where a seemingly humble tuber silently sculpted societal shifts. The introduction of the potato not only brought about agricultural and nutritional transformations but also subtly chiseled at the social structures, providing sustenance during famines and enabling populations to thrive, altering labor patterns and societal demographics.

Sustainable Societies of Indigenous Peoples

As our journey winds, we observe indigenous societies worldwide, where sustenance was harvested in harmony with nature, and food distribution echoed the values of egalitarianism and communal living. From the Iroquois Confederacy practicing sustainable agriculture to the nomadic Maasai, whose cattle-centric livelihoods pulsated with cultural and societal significance, the echoes of their food practices reverberate through time, whispering tales of sustainability and social cohesion.

In each morsel of food, there lies a narrative far more extensive and intricate than one might presume. The societal structures and the philosophies underpinning them have always been, in numerous ways, sculpted by the choices, practices, and, often, the politics of food.

In this chapter, as we simmered through various civilizations, we've tasted not just the flavors but also sensed the undercurrents of societal norms, upheavals, and evolutions stirred by food. Our quest is far from over, dear reader. With bellies and minds slightly fuller, let's continue to feast on the bountiful histories and stories served up by the past, exploring further how the culinary can be cultural, political, and societal, all simmering in a pot of complex, yet nourishing stew of civilization.

14

PREHISTORIC CULINARY INNOVATIONS

It's hard to believe that our distant ancestors, unacquainted with the modern kitchen's hums and beeps, could be culinary innovators. But oh, how they were! Today's chapter unfolds the tale of gastronomy where cookbooks were unheard of, and the kitchen was the boundless wild.

Rock, Fire, and Bone Tools: The First Culinary Implements

In the absence of blenders, food processors, and fancy knives, our prehistoric forebears turned to nature's pantry. Rocks became pounding tools, and the discovery of fire was akin to unboxing the first oven! They meticulously cracked, crushed, and cooked, unwittingly laying down the first chapters of culinary arts.

Imagine the magic of tasting cooked meat for the first time, its tenderness and enhanced flavors, a stark contrast to the regular raw morsels. Fire didn't only warm them amidst the chilly prehistoric nights but opened a whole new world of gastronomy!

Fermentation: The Ancient Alchemist

Fermentation must have seemed like an enchanting sorcery back then. Picture this: A forgotten pouch of gathered grains gets wet, days pass, and voilà, the first beer is accidentally brewed! This unintentional discovery of fermentation was not merely a delightful surprise but a significant culinary milestone, preserving food, enhancing nutritional value, and, well, making parties a bit more lively!

Stone Age Sushi and Ocean Delights

Journey to the Jōmon period in ancient Japan, where folks had mastered the art of fishing with hooks made from the jagged fragments of sea shells. Think of it as the inception of sushi, as they paired fresh fish with fermented rice, creating a primitive version of a delicacy that has swum its way through millennia to our contemporary sushi bars.

Herbs and Spices: The Primitive Palate Explorers

Our ancestors, albeit with a simpler toolkit, were sophisticated in their understanding of flora and fauna, identifying which berries sweetened their meals and which herbs healed their ailments. They became the original flavor explorers, experimenting with various herbs and spices, infusing their food with bursts of flavors we continue to cherish today.

The Original Slow Cooking

We also owe the art of slow cooking to our ancient foremothers and forefathers. They discovered that burying food in the embers of a fire and allowing it to cook slowly not only preserved the nutrition but also tenderized tougher cuts of meat, providing an unanticipated luxury in their otherwise harsh and survival-driven lives.

Pottery: Unlocking New Culinary Doors

And then came pottery – a simple innovation that unleashed an array of culinary possibilities! No longer was cooking confined to skewering and roasting. Now, foods could be boiled, stewed, and stored, unlocking a plethora of flavors and techniques.

A Foraging Lifestyle: Earth's Bountiful Pantry

Gathering wasn't merely about sustenance but an intimate understanding and respect for nature's rhythms. They knew when berries ripened, which mushrooms to relish and which to avoid, and where the juiciest roots nestled underground. This symbiotic relationship with nature not only enriched their diet but embedded sustainability into their everyday lives.

From crackling fires of ancient times to our modern stovetops, from stone tools to stainless steel, the culinary journey has been nothing short of spectacular. Today, as we scrutinize our dishes, may we remember the ancestral hands that crafted the first meals, their experiments, their innovations, and the simplicity that sired complexity.

They may not have had our technologies, but our prehistoric ancestors had a boundless, beautiful environment that was both a home and a haven of culinary wonders. As we travel forth into the subsequent chapters, we keep their spirit of innovation and exploration alight, navigating through the evolving epochs of gastronomy, with a dash of appreciation and a sprinkle of curiosity, forever entwining our contemporary kitchens with the ancient fires that once flickered under prehistoric pots.

15

SPICES, TRADE, AND GLOBAL PALATES

We're embarking on a zesty adventure through time, where the pursuit of flavors whisked humanity across vast oceans and uncharted territories. Our 15th chapter, dear reader, is an aromatic journey through the entwining trails of spices, trade, and the evolution of our global palates.

A Dash of Spice: Transforming Meals and Economies

Intricate networks of ancient trade routes, like veins, pulsed with commodities that bound distant lands in a tight web of economic and culinary exchange. Pepper, cinnamon, cloves, and myriad exotic aromas wafted through the docks of ancient ports, whispering of far-off lands and adventures to every passerby.

These weren't just condiments; they were nuggets of gold, altering not just the flavors but the very socio-economic tides of the regions they touched. Spices were not merely culinary enhancers; they were preservatives, medicines, and symbols of status.

The Fragrant Silk Road

The Silk Road, renowned for its role in connecting the East and West, wasn't just a highway for silks and jewels but a bustling avenue where culinary secrets were whispered across continents. It was where the warmth of Indian spices met the subtlety of Chinese teas and where Mediterranean olive oil kissed the rich textures of Central Asian nuts and dried fruits.

Imagine the first European noble, tasting pepper for the first time, an explosion of unfamiliar yet enticing heat playing upon his palate, forever enchanting him with the mystique of the East.

Turbulent Seas and Spicy Ventures

Daring voyages undertaken by sailors like Columbus and Vasco da Gama were not merely quests for new lands but a pursuit for the aromatic and the zesty, which had become as valuable as precious metals. These journeys were perilous, yet the allure of spices propelled explorations, discoveries, and eventually, unexpected culinary fusions.

Colonialism: A Bitter Aftertaste

Yet, this tapestry of spice and trade also weaves a tale of exploitation and oppression. Colonial powers, intoxicated by the wealth promised by spice islands and trade routes, perpetuated brutalities and subjugation in their quest to dominate the spice trade. It's essential to honor the stories of indigenous communities who were eclipsed by the shadow of colonial aspirations and to remember that many favored spices have a bitter history.

The Melting Pot of Global Cuisine

Despite the darkness that sometimes marred the spice trade, it also unintentionally facilitated a culinary melting pot. Imagine Italian cuisine without the sweet tang of tomatoes, originally native to the Americas, or Indian delicacies without the potent punch of chili, which also hailed from the New World.

Spices and trade have knit a colorful quilt of flavors, where ingredients native to one corner of the globe found new homes in distant lands, forging the dynamic, multicultural palette of global cuisine we relish today.

An Aromatic Future

As we swirl our modern-day curries and sprinkle spices onto our dishes, we engage in a ritual that has bound humanity through millennia. Today, as we stand in an era where any spice is but a click away, we must ponder upon the pathways of the past and envisage a future that honors sustainability, fairness, and ethical practices in our culinary adventures.

The Spice Route's Legacy: Culinary Evolution

Let's pause and delve into the contemporary kitchens, shall we? Even today, if we trace back the essence of our beloved dishes, we can see the intricate fingerprints of ancestral trade routes. The simmering Bolognese sauce, the aromatic Indian curry, or the comforting bowl of Vietnamese pho – each a potpourri of flavors, curated from various corners of our vibrant world.

Our ancestors, albeit unknowingly, crafted today's culinary tapestry by intertwining their local flavors with those from distant lands, learned through tales told by weary travelers, spirited traders, and adventurous explorers.

Unwrapping Culinary Packets: Tamales to Dumplings

Dive deep with me into an unexpected beneficiary of the spice trade: our beloved little food packets! From the spicy tamales of Mesoamerica, steamy Chinese dumplings, to the rich, hearty Cornish pasties of England, these delightful parcels spell comfort in every cuisine. They traverse cultures and epochs, showcasing a delightful meld of local ingredients and introduced flavors, narrating tales of trade, migration, and culinary innovation.

Savoring Sustainability: An Age-Old Tradition

Reflect on the indigenous communities, who, despite the ebb and flow of empires and the rush of spice traders, have sustained their culinary traditions, tethering them like anchors to their cultural identity. Their symbiotic relationship with their environment, a rich tapestry of sustainable practices, continues to awe and inspire chefs and food enthusiasts worldwide.

For them, every herb, root, and spice isn't merely a flavor enhancer but a potent reminder of their ethos, wherein nature isn't exploited but embraced, honored, and preserved.

The Spice in Modern Times: A Nod to the Past, A Look to the Future

Today, while we enjoy an eclectic array of cuisines, seasoned with spices sourced from every nook and cranny of our planet, it's vital to reminisce about the journeys endured by each fragrant granule. From being the currency of the affluent to becoming a staple on our shelves, spices have traversed a path that's deeply intertwined with our societal and culinary evolution.

As we step into an era that's returning to its roots, seeking sustainability, fairness, and ethical practices, the story of spices unfolds not just as a historical chapter but as a guide, echoing the lessons, mistakes, and triumphs of our predecessors.

Seasoning the Future: Your Role in the Culinary Saga

And here you are, dear reader, a pivotal character in the ongoing saga of spices and culinary adventures. As you sprinkle cinnamon on your morning oatmeal or add a dash of cayenne to your evening stew, remember: you're continuing a tradition that has been alive for millennia.

As you explore global cuisines, recognize not merely the flavors but the histories, the tales of love, war, and exploration that have seeped into every grain and every leaf. And, as you concoct your culinary creations, may you also weave a story that future generations will savor, one of respect for all cultures and sustainable stewardship of our planet's bountiful pantry.

And thus, the savory scents of the spice-laden breeze gently nudge us into the upcoming chapters. As we unfurl more tales of culinary adventures through the annals of time, let's carry forward the rich, complex, and sometimes poignant histories that have shaped our meals and our worlds.

16

LESSONS FROM EXTINCT CULTURES AND CIVILIZATIONS

Have you ever paused for a moment, while biting into a crisp apple or sipping a fragrant tea, and wondered what culinary marvels delighted the palates of those in ancient, now-extinct civilizations? Chapter 16 invites us on a fantastical journey to explore the culinary worlds of civilizations that once bloomed, showcasing rich, vibrant cultures, only to silently retreat back into the sands of time, leaving behind mystifying relics and enchanting tales.

A Stroll Through the Magnificent Maya

Let's step into the lush, verdant world of the Mayans, a civilization that flourished with astounding astronomical, architectural, and culinary prowess. Imagine strolling through their bustling markets, where vibrant cacao beans were not just ingredients but currency. The Mayans, with their profound understanding of their natural environment, concocted the precursor to our beloved chocolate, a frothy, chili-infused beverage that was realms apart from the sweet, creamy concoction we adore today.

Their cuisine, a splendid melange of maize, beans, chili peppers, and an assortment of fruits, provides a splendid lens through which we can perceive their connectivity and harmony with the land they inhabited.

Savoring the Sophistication of Sumer

Now, let's traverse to the fertile crescent of Mesopotamia, where the Sumerians, with their cuneiform writings and ziggurats, sowed the seeds for future generations to reap the benefits of organized agriculture and societal structures. Their meals, often a hearty blend of barley, onions, and leeks, cooked into stews with meats and dried fruits, mirror their structured societal and agricultural systems, revealing their knack for coordination and collective effort.

The Sumerians also held beer in high regard, a beverage that was consumed by both adults and children, symbolizing not just their brewing capabilities but also their comprehension of fermentation processes.

Unlocking Culinary Secrets of the Indus Valley

Shifting our gaze towards the sophisticated Indus Valley civilization, we discover a society that thrived on agricultural abundance and well-planned urban establishments. Their granaries, which stand testament to their bountiful harvests and efficient storage systems, whisper tales of a diet that was predominantly vegetarian, reliant on wheat, barley, and a multitude of vegetables.

Imagine the aroma wafting through their kitchens as they prepared flatbreads, perhaps flavored with the now globally-renowned spices like cumin and coriander, offering us a subtle hint towards India's spice-dominated culinary journey.

A Respectful Nod to the Enigmatic Rapa Nui

Let's then sail to the remote Easter Island, where the Rapa Nui civilization, renowned for their giant, stoic Moai statues, prompts us to ponder upon the precarious balance between human ingenuity and environmental sustainability. Their story, which perhaps pivots around overexploitation of resources, encourages us to reflect upon our current relationship with our planet and its offerings.

Each of these extinct civilizations, through their culinary practices and agricultural methodologies, unfolds a chapter that melds human innovation, societal structures, and the perpetual dance with nature's bounty.

Why We Must Listen to These Culinary Echoes from the Past

What might appear as mere historical tales actually hold the keys to understanding the intertwining of culture, environment, and cuisine. The silent stories encrypted in the ruins of these civilizations resonate with lessons of sustainability, respect for natural resources, and the essentiality of harmonious coexistence with our environment.

Unraveling the Flavors of the Ancient Egyptians

As we saunter further along our journey, we come to the sun-drenched banks of the Nile, where the ancient Egyptians, renowned for their pyramids and prolific philosophical advancements, left behind inscriptions and artifacts that illuminate their culinary culture. Imagine the richness of a civilization that meticulously planned afterlives while simultaneously ensuring life itself was vibrant and flavorful.

Ancient Egyptians weren't merely builders of the magnificent pyramids; they were connoisseurs of bread and beer, staples that reverberated through all strata of society. The ample wheat and barley fields alongside the Nile not only yielded their daily bread but also fermented into a myriad of beer variations. Their baking and brewing weren't just about sustenance but were interwoven with their religious beliefs and societal interactions.

Picture the bustling marketplaces where dates, figs, and grapes were traded vigorously, later to be transformed into sweet delicacies and fermented into wines, revealing the ancient Egyptian's refined palate and their ability to manipulate natural resources to serve their culinary and societal needs.

An Ode to the Anasazi and Their Enigmatic End

Journeying to the rugged terrains of the American Southwest, we encounter the vestiges of the Anasazi, or the Ancient Puebloans. This enigmatic civilization, credited with constructing the intricate cliff dwellings, also wove a culinary narrative deeply embedded in the harsh, arid environment they called home.

They weren't merely survivalists but culinary innovators, manipulating corn – their lifeblood – into a variety of sustenance forms. The Anasazi cultivated beans and squash, practicing an early form of sustainable agriculture, crafting a diet that was incredibly harmonious with the challenging landscape.

Yet, as we gaze upon the hauntingly abandoned cliff palaces, we're prompted to contemplate their abrupt disappearance. Does their mystery laden departure whisper warnings to our contemporary civilizations about the fragility of societies in the face of environmental changes?

Discovering the Resilient Scythians

Venturing into the vast steppes of Eurasia, we encounter the nomadic Scythians, warriors renowned for their horsemanship and detailed gold work. Much of what we infer about their culinary culture comes from the tombs, encapsulating not just bodies but a snapshot of their dietary and ritualistic practices.

Meat, particularly that of horses, played a pivotal role, revealing a diet heavily reliant on pastoral practices. The Scythians navigated through extremes, from battling harsh winters to managing vast herds across extensive terrains, their dietary practices echoing a life that was perpetually on the move and attuned to the cycles of nature.

Reflections and Forward Movements

While these ancient tales and mysterious extinctions may seem distant and shrouded in bygone eras, they are undeniably intertwined with our present-day culinary practices and globalized food systems. Their innovative cooking methods, the ingredients they cherished, and their societal structures forged around food production and consumption are not merely historical anecdotes but are threads woven into the vast, intricate tapestry of our collective culinary heritage.

As we muse upon these past civilizations and their intricate relationships with food, we find ourselves standing at a pivotal juncture where our actions, choices, and respect towards our environment and food sources will inscribe our chapter in history.

In the chapters to follow, we shall delve into how modern societies can glean wisdom from these ancient practices, ensuring that our culinary future is sustainable, vibrant, and most importantly, in harmony with the planet that continually nourishes us.

17

WILD VS. FARMED: ANALYZING THE DICHOTOMY

As our path through the dense forests of historical culinary wisdom unfolds, let's embark on a chapter that sets the stage for an age-old debate that reverberates through our dietary choices even today: the dichotomy between wild and farmed foods.

The Raw Allure of the Wild

Let's journey first into the wild, where nature lays out a banquet unrestricted by fences or furrows. The very essence of wild foods lies in their untamed nature, sprouting, blooming, and thriving amidst the diverse ecosystems, unswayed by human hands. Picture the hunter-gatherers, our ancestors, who roamed vast expanses with a discerning eye and honed instincts, foraging for berries, mushrooms, and nuts, while hunting game that grazed on nature's unbridled bounty.

Wild foods are not merely ingredients; they are tales of seasons, ecosystems, and the complex web of life. A single wild berry is a culmination of the interplay between sunlight, soil, rain, and myriad life forms, offering not just sustenance but a connection to the pulsating life that surrounds it.

Sown Seeds and the Birth of Agriculture

As our footsteps tread from the wild terrains into organized farmlands, we witness the evolution from merely consuming what nature offers, to curating, and controlling what and how food is grown. Here, seeds carefully sown transform into neatly arranged rows of crops, providing a reliable, predictable bounty at each harvest.

The introduction of farming catapulted humanity into civilizations, ushering in a newfound stability that permitted us to lay down roots, both literally and metaphorically. Crops like wheat, rice, and maize became not just staples but the very bedrock upon which societies were built, shaping our culinary and cultural landscapes in profound ways.

A Delicate Balance: Wild and Farmed Coexistence

While the reliability of farming has undeniable merits, can we overlook the allure and nutritional diversity that wild foods offer? The wild, with its uncharted terrains and unscripted bounty, whispers tales of diversity and survival, while the farmed assures us with its stability and predictability.

Can the lush wild forests coexist with the neatly demarcated fields? Our ancestors foraged and farmed, oscillating between the wild and the cultivated, crafting a diet that was both diverse and reliable.

Bridging the Divide with Culinary Wisdom

Imagine, for a moment, a plate that honors both these worlds, marrying the predictability of farmed grains with the adventurous spirit of wild greens. Can the stabilizing essence of agriculture be infused with the robust, diverse flavors of the wild?

Perhaps, within this dichotomy lies the potential for a diet that is not just sustainable and nourishing but also inherently respectful of the planet that hosts us. Within this mingling of wild and farmed, we might find culinary practices that celebrate not just the food but the myriad life forms, ecosystems, and elements that bring these ingredients to our tables.

And this, dear reader, brings us to a juncture where the chapters ahead will delve deeper into how we, the modern inhabitants of this ancient, timeless planet, can weave together the wild and the farmed into our culinary tapestry.

18

THE POWER OF PLANT-BASED EATING IN ANTIQUITY

Our collective gastronomic journey through times yore now brings us to the lush and verdant world of plant-based eating in antiquity. Isn't it fascinating to think about how our forebears understood, even then, the incredible power housed within roots, leaves, seeds, and fruits?

A Blossoming Respect for Flora

In ancient times, plants were not just recognized for their nutritional value but were embedded in the very essence of cultures. Let's imagine ourselves strolling through the gardens of Babylon, where the air was scented with fragrant herbs and where fruits hung plentifully, a testament to the ancient wisdom that recognized the potent power of plants.

Here, in these terraced wonders, plants were more than sustenance; they were medicines, ritualistic elements, and even symbols of prosperity and power. It wasn't merely about consuming plants but understanding them, knowing when to sow and when to reap, understanding which plant could heal and which could harm.

The Plant-Based Diets of Ancient Civilizations

Picture, if you will, the tables of ancient Greece, where philosophers like Pythagoras touted the merits of a plant-based diet, intertwining ethics, health, and spirituality into their eating habits. Vegetables, legumes, fruits, and grains were not merely side dishes but the very essence of meals, prepared with a simplicity that allowed the natural flavors to shine, often seasoned only with a dash of olive oil and fragrant herbs.

And let us journey further east, to the vibrant landscapes of ancient India, where the roots of vegetarianism were deeply entwined with philosophical and spiritual beliefs. Here, the concept of 'Ahimsa' or non-violence extended to dietary practices, culminating in meals that were a melange of colors, flavors, and textures, all derived from the plant kingdom.

The Confluence of Nourishment and Respect

Peering back into these historical snippets, there is an evident reverence towards the plant kingdom, recognizing their crucial role in sustaining life and ensuring health. These ancient civilizations, through observation and understanding, unearthed the secret that plants could nourish them without necessitating harm to other beings.

This plant-based wisdom was not merely about abstaining from meat but about embracing the boundless variety and potential that plants offered. It was about understanding the rhythms of nature, respecting the cycles of growth and decay, and aligning dietary practices harmoniously with these natural ebbs and flows.

Seeds of Thought for Modern Days

What can we, ensconced in our modern worlds, glean from these ancient practices of plant-based eating? There's an unspoken beauty and wisdom in recognizing the power that plants hold, not merely as a source of sustenance but as entities that sustain life in all its myriad forms.

This chapter is not just a historical jaunt but a seed sown for contemplation about how our dietary choices echo through time, influencing our health, societies, and the very planet that cradles us. As we turn the pages ahead, let's carry forward this ancestral knowledge, pondering upon how we can reincorporate this timeless wisdom into our contemporary plates and lives.

SECTION II

Global Plates: A Journey Through Culinary Cultures

19

THE SPICE ROUTES AND CULINARY EXCHANGE

In our comforting kitchens, we casually sprinkle cinnamon, black pepper, and nutmeg onto our dishes, perhaps not pondering the immense journeys these spices have embarked upon throughout history.

Navigating Through the Spice Routes

Allow me to whisk you away to a time where the earth was still a mystery and the known world was a patchwork of kingdoms and empires, vibrant and diverse. It was the allure of spices, with their captivating aromas and transformative flavors, that nudged brave souls to venture into the unknown, stitching a thread that would weave together the culinary tapestries of diverse cultures.

The ancient spice routes, be it the maritime paths caressed by the sea or the overland trails tread by camel feet, were not merely routes of trade but avenues through which knowledge, culture, and culinary wisdom permeated distant lands. Imagine, a simple black pepper corn traveling thousands of miles, across tumultuous seas and arid deserts, to find itself in a distant kitchen, transforming local dishes with its exotic warmth.

A Melting Pot of Flavors and Cultures

This journey is not merely about the movement of goods, but about the intermingling of ideas, philosophies, and culinary traditions. The cinnamon from the exotic East did not only spice up the European stews but brought with it whispers of faraway lands, of empires that basked in the golden sun and of forests where trees bled fragrant resins.

In reverse, imagine the Indian curry, adapting and evolving as it meandered through the spice route, absorbing the culinary influences of the Middle Eastern merchants, the Central Asian nomads, and the European sailors.

The Spice: A Symbol of Unity and Diversity

As we delve deeper into the tales from the spice route, it is enchanting to perceive spices not merely as commodities but as bearers of stories, of ancient secrets, and of the unity that exists within our diverse culinary landscapes.

The cloves that simmer in our soups are the same that were once used to preserve meats in medieval Europe, to enhance the flavors of imperial Chinese teas, and to scent the homes of the ancient Romans. The cumin that adds a warm depth to our stews also wafted through the bazaars of ancient Alexandria, lingered in the royal kitchens of Persia, and was cherished in the courts of the Indian Maharajas.

The Modern Plate: A Mosaic of Ancient Routes

Our plates today are, perhaps unbeknownst to us, a vibrant mosaic crafted through centuries of exchange, exploration, and shared culinary wisdom. The tomatoes of the Americas salsa-dancing through Italian pasta, the fiery chillies of Mexico lighting up Korean kimchi, and the fragrant basil of Asia adding its fresh kiss to a Greek salad—these are all testaments to our interconnected global palate.

As we explore the depths of the chapters ahead, let's savor each flavor, each story, and each fragment of knowledge, recognizing that our modern culinary landscapes are rich tapestries woven through centuries of global exchange, adventure, and shared humanity.

20

FEASTING AND FASTING: CULTURAL PERSPECTIVES

As we delve into the worlds of feasting and fasting, we immerse ourselves into the profound duality that has, for centuries, shaped the culinary and cultural landscapes across the globe.

Feasting: A Symphony of Abundance

When we talk about feasts, what swirls into your mind? Perhaps tables laden with platters of rich, decadent food, the air punctuated with laughter, and a melody of chatters and cheers? Feasts, in their myriad forms, have always been more than a mere assembly of dishes. They are a spectacle where food becomes the medium through which joy, gratitude, and camaraderie are expressed.

From the lavish banquets of ancient Rome to the opulent feasts of the Mughal emperors, these occasions of abundance were as much about showcasing culinary prowess and wealth as they were about celebrating, sharing, and expressing generosity.

But let's peer a bit closer and ponder: is a feast merely about abundance?

Fasting: The Profound Silence of Plates

Contrastingly, we wander into the realms of fasting, where the absence of food echoes with a different kind of abundance - spiritual, mental, and physical purification. Fasting, in its essence, isn't just a denial of food but a time of reflection, a period where the body and spirit are cleansed, and where one retreats inward, whether for religious beliefs, health reasons, or societal practices.

From the solemnity of the Ramadan fast to the reflective period of Lent, fasting has boundlessly permeated global cultures, each bringing forth its own philosophies and practices related to abstaining. Here, the quiet of the empty plate whispers tales of discipline, devotion, and contemplation.

A Dance of Polarities

Feasting and fasting might seem like polar opposites, yet they are entwined in a perpetual dance, where each gives meaning and context to the other. The feast gains its value through the backdrop of everyday moderation or periods of fasting, while the fast is given depth and anticipation through the celebratory lens of the feasts that may break it.

This duality encompasses a universal truth that pervades culinary cultures across the world: the balance of excess and restraint, celebration and contemplation, indulgence and discipline.

Tales of Feasts and Fasts

As we weave through the narratives of various cultures and their practices of feasting and fasting in the chapters ahead, we'll explore not merely the foods that grace and absent from their tables, but the profound meanings, philosophies, and traditions that envelop these practices.

Join me, will you, as we embark upon a journey that will take us through time and across continents, exploring the resonances of feasts and fasts that have for centuries, defined, and been defined by, the societal, spiritual, and cultural structures of civilizations.

21 REGIONAL STAPLES AND THEIR CULTURAL SIGNIFICANCE

Today, we journey across terrains and traverse through diverse cultures, exploring the humble, yet profoundly significant, regional staples that have sustained and shaped civilizations. The very backbone of myriad cuisines, these staples whisper tales of survival, tradition, and culinary innovation.

The Humble Rice Grain

Let's meander through the lush, verdant paddy fields of Asia, where a single grain of rice is a droplet of life itself. In its delicate husk, rice carries generations of agricultural, culinary, and cultural history. From the ceremonial sake of Japan to the aromatic biryanis of India, rice is not merely sustenance but a symbol of life, prosperity, and celebration.

Corn: The Golden Gift of the Americas

Sailing across to the vibrant landscapes of the Americas, we encounter corn, standing tall and regal in its golden splendor. The ancient Mayans revered it, the Native Americans celebrated it, and the modern world savors it in its myriad forms, from tortillas to polenta. Corn, in its varied avatars, unfolds narratives of discovery, colonization, and cultural synthesis.

Wheat: Sowing the Seeds of Civilizations

Now, wander with me through the expansive wheat fields that gently sway in the European and Middle Eastern breezes. Bread, in its countless forms, from the robust loaves of Germany to the soft, embracing pita of the Levant, tells stories of communities, of families gathering around tables, sharing meals, stories, and forming bonds that have withstood the sands of time.

The Resilient Cassava

Diving into the rich, warm soils of Africa, we find the roots of sustenance buried deep within – the cassava. A crop of resilience and versatility, cassava has whispered to its farmers tales of endurance, providing nourishment in climates harsh and unforgiving. From fluffy fufu to crispy tapioca, cassava brings to the table a rich array of dishes that form the heartbeat of numerous African cuisines.

Potatoes: From the Andes to the World

Climb with me, atop the majestic Andean ranges, where the humble potato was unearthed. A tuber that voyaged across oceans, permeating kitchens worldwide, transforming cuisines and shaping histories. Whether in an Irish stew, a Belgian fry, or an Indian curry, the potato, modest and unassuming, silently weaves tales of globalization, famine, and culinary innovation.

Journeying Through Tales of Staple Foods

These staples, each with their own unique tales of journey and transformation, have been more than mere ingredients; they have been silent witnesses to human history, shaping and being shaped by the hands that have sown, harvested, and cooked them.

As we saunter through the pages ahead, immersing ourselves into the stories, recipes, and traditions surrounding these regional staples, we shall explore not just the physical journey of seeds, roots, and grains, but the cultural, spiritual, and emotional imprints they have left upon civilizations.

22

THE SOCIOLOGY OF FOOD AND EATING HABITS

In this chapter, we're going to unwrap the fascinating enigma that entwines the sociology of food with our everyday lives. This isn't merely a story about what's on our plates but a heartening delve into how what we eat entwines with our social fabric.

The Shared Table: More Than a Meal

Let's begin with the quintessential act of eating together. Whether it's a family gathering around a homely dinner or friends clinking glasses over a sumptuous spread, the act of sharing a meal is deeply embedded in our social conduct. The Italian pranzo, a midday meal, is not just about savoring delightful flavors; it's a robust, lingering event, where conversations flow as smoothly as the wine. Meanwhile, the American Thanksgiving, with its iconic turkey and stuffing, is not merely a feast but a symbol of gratitude, sharing, and familial bonds.

Status on a Plate: Culinary Social Markers

Ever pondered how our culinary choices become reflections, even declarations, of our social status and identity? Consider the illustrious French truffle or the luxurious Japanese kobe beef. These aren't simply ingredients; they are symbols, whispering tales of luxury, exclusivity, and a certain social standing. Whereas, staples like rice, beans, and potatoes, each with their own rich history, often speak to the masses, anchoring cuisines and cultures in a shared, communal experience.

Religion, Ethics, and Plates

Journeying through global plates, we witness how religious and ethical beliefs seamlessly blend into culinary traditions. The vegetarian thalis of India, not merely vibrant in flavors but also embodying a spiritual and philosophical ethos. Kosher and halal practices, intertwining faith and food, guide not just what is consumed but how it's prepared and eaten. And then, the growing vegan movement, reflecting not merely a dietary choice but a stance on environmental ethics and animal welfare.

Politics, Power, and Pastries

Ah, and let's not forget how food has played a pivotal role in political narratives. French Revolution, anyone? When the peasants were told, "Let them eat cake," the subtle undercurrents of food distribution, accessibility, and class disparities were laid bare. Food has often been the symbol and medium of power dynamics, control, and resistance across societies.

Gender and Culinary Spaces

As we sift through culinary tales, we encounter the gendered spaces within culinary worlds. Often, professional kitchens have been masculinized, with the stereotype of the authoritative male chef reigning supreme. Contrast this with the domestic sphere, where women have traditionally been the nurturers, cooking for their families, and you unveil a rich dialogue on gender, power, and space within the culinary domain.

Food as Cultural Identity

And then, we navigate through the heartening stories where food becomes a steadfast symbol of cultural identity and continuity, especially amongst diasporic communities. The poignant tales of immigrants, where the flavors of home provide comfort, continuity, and a tangible connection to their roots, present a vivid tableau of how food becomes a silent, yet potent, carrier of identity, memory, and heritage.

In this delicious chapter, our exploration into the sociology of food invites us to perceive our culinary practices not just as mere acts of consumption but as meaningful rituals, woven intricately into our social, religious, and cultural tapestries. So, let's continue to feast on the rich, layered stories that unfold in the chapters ahead, exploring the diverse culinary landscapes that our beautiful world has to offer. Our exploration is as boundless as our appetite is insatiable – onwards, fellow culinary explorers, to the next flavorful adventure!

23
EUROPEAN CULINARY EVOLUTION

Welcome back to our epicurean journey through time and culture. Today, let's embark on a fascinating exploration of a continent where culinary artistry is woven into the very fabric of its culture: Europe.

In the Beginning: A Rich Agricultural Bounty

Europe, with its bounteous fields, fertile valleys, and abundant waters, has been a haven for agricultural innovation since time immemorial. The early Europeans, with their rich offerings of grains, legumes, and livestock, carved out a dietary path that flowed from necessity to sophistication. Cereals were converted into hearty bread, legumes transformed into hearty stews, and fruits were preserved as delightful jams, becoming staples upon the European table.

The Medieval Melting Pot

As we traverse into the medieval era, we uncover a blend of eclectic flavors, with spices like pepper, cinnamon, and ginger embarking on a piquant journey across the continent via complex trade routes. Kings and peasants alike reveled in the newfound complexity that these ingredients brought to their meals. Elaborate feasts with roasted meats, aromatic pies, and sweetmeats adorned the tables of the wealthy, while simple, hearty, and nourishing meals prevailed amidst the working class.

Renaissance: A Culinary Rebirth

The Renaissance brought not only a revival of art and literature but also an innovative spirit that spilled into the kitchen. Cookery was elevated to an art form, where chefs began to experiment with flavors, techniques, and presentations. Ingredients like tomatoes, potatoes, and chocolate, discovered from the New World, gradually entwined themselves into the European culinary narrative, crafting a new chapter in its gastronomic history.

The French Culinary Beacon

Ah, when discussing European culinary art, how can we omit the French with their exquisite sauces, delicate pastries, and culinary techniques that have shaped the global culinary scene? France, with its meticulous attention to flavor, technique, and presentation, established itself as a gastronomic epicenter, influencing chefs and gourmands across borders and generations.

The Homely Charm of Italian Cuisine

Now, imagine the warmth of an Italian kitchen, where nonna kneads her dough for the perfect pasta, where ripe tomatoes, fragrant basil, and rich olive oil meld into a symphony of flavors. Italian cuisine, with its heartwarming simplicity, robust flavors, and regional diversity, has enamored palates worldwide, telling tales of its land and people through every bite.

The Versatility of Spanish Flavors

And then, there's Spain, with its vibrant tapas culture, the rich, smoky aroma of paprika, and the comforting consistency of paella, crafting a culinary tapestry that's diverse, spirited, and heartening. Whether sipping on a sultry sangria or savoring a spicy chorizo, the

Spanish showcase a delightful balance between traditional and innovative culinary artistry.

Exploring Beyond: A Melange of Flavors

Of course, European cuisine is not just defined by these powerhouse nations. From the hearty sausages of Germany, the elegant chocolates of Belgium, to the earthy, hearty flavors of Slavic cuisine, Europe offers a delightful mosaic of tastes, textures, and traditions, each nation contributing its unique note to this harmonious symphony.

24
A TASTE OF ASIA: TRADITION VS. MODERNITY

Buckle up, for today we cast our nets over the colossal and immensely diverse continent of Asia, where tradition and modernity beautifully interweave to create a gastronomic tapestry unlike any other. From the aromatic spice bazaars of India to the bustling night markets of Taiwan, we're about to explore a culinary realm that's boundlessly rich and thrillingly varied.

Bowing to Tradition: The Root of Asian Cuisine

At the heart of Asian cuisine lies a profound respect for tradition. Picture this: a Japanese sushi master meticulously crafting each nigiri, with years of precision training guiding every delicate slice. Or consider the Indian "masalchis" (spice mixers), who blend an array of spices into masalas that have flavored the nation's dishes for centuries. These culinary practices, deeply rooted in tradition, have not only survived but thrived amidst the rapid modernization across the continent.

The Spice Route: A Trail of Aromas and Flavors

Embarking on the historic Spice Route, we traverse through lands where cloves, nutmeg, cardamom, and pepper were once considered more valuable than gold. In India, these spices are not merely ingredients but symbols of the country's colorful, vibrant culture. Every pinch of turmeric and cumin tells a tale, not just enhancing the dish but whispering ancient stories through each bite.

The Rice Bowl: Essential Grain, Varied Traditions

Rice, a staple that has nourished billions across Asia, presents itself in mesmerizingly diverse forms as we journey from one region to another. From the delicate sushi rice of Japan, the aromatic basmati of India, to the sticky rice dumplings of China – rice is not just sustenance but a canvas through which various Asian cultures express their culinary identity and creativity.

Street Food: A Symphony of Chaos and Flavors

Ah, the bustling, vibrant street food scenes of Asia! Picture Thailand's vivacious markets where sizzling woks toss together a lively Pad Thai, or the Vietnamese stalls lining the streets of Hanoi, with simmering pots of pho awaiting eager diners. Street food, with its unpretentious, authentic, and incredibly flavorful offerings, represents a culinary arena where the age-old and the contemporary deliciously collide.

Fine Dining and Modern Twists

Asia also elegantly embraces the modern without letting go of the traditional. Picture contemporary Indian or Chinese restaurants where age-old recipes meet innovative techniques, resulting in a delightful culinary hybrid that pays homage to the past while nodding to the future. Singapore, with its spectacular array of Michelin-starred restaurants, epitomizes this marriage of the old and the new, offering a culinary experience that's luxurious, innovative, yet steeped in tradition.

Regional Diversity: A Culinary Kaleidoscope

Asia, with its staggering regional diversity, offers a never-ending culinary adventure. The fiery, wok-tossed delights of Sichuan, the fragrant curries of Kerala, the robust, hearty flavors of Korean barbecue – each region, with its unique ingredients, techniques, and flavors, contributes to the dazzlingly complex culinary quilt that is distinctly Asian.

And so, dear readers, as we saunter through the scintillating streets of Asia, we observe a marvelous dance between the ancient and the modern, where recipes passed down through generations seamlessly blend with contemporary tastes and techniques, crafting a culinary narrative that's extraordinarily rich, endlessly diverse, and tantalizingly delicious.

25

THE RICHNESS OF AFRICAN CULINARY HERITAGE

A realm where millennia-old culinary traditions intertwine with innovative modern techniques, Africa presents a fascinating mosaic of flavors, textures, and aromas that span from the sun-soaked Mediterranean coasts to the lush, vibrant heartlands of the sub-Saharan.

The Pan-African Palate: A Vast Culinary Expedition

African cuisine, although spoken of in a singular term, is far from a monolithic entity. Each region, each nation, and indeed, each community presents its distinct culinary paradigm. From the spice-laden dishes of the North, marked by Arab and Mediterranean influences, to the maize-based staples of the South – the culinary landscape is as varied as it is vast.

Communal Dining: The African Way

Picture the wide, welcoming smiles and outstretched hands, inviting you to partake in a communal feast, a prevalent and culturally significant dining style across many African societies. The notion of 'Ubuntu', an Nguni Bantu term translating to 'humanity', reflects abundantly in the eating habits. Meals are not merely about nourishment but are a binding thread that fortifies relationships, communities, and cultures.

Roots, Tubers, and Grains: The Sustaining Staples

Venturing through the labyrinth of African gastronomy, we encounter a spectacular array of staples - from yams and cassava to millets and teff. In Nigeria, behold the majestic 'Pounded Yam' and Egusi soup, a melodious blend of yam flour, melon seeds, leafy vegetables, and meat, embodying a perfect harmony of flavors and textures.

Spices and Aromas: Painting with Nature's Palette

The African spice palette is extravagantly colorful and aromatically enchanting. Think of Ethiopian Berbere, a fiery, fragrant blend that breathes life into stews and meats. Or consider Ras el Hanout from Morocco, a delicate, aromatic symphony that whispers the secrets of ancient spice routes into every dish it graces.

Street Foods: A Gastronomic Adventure on Every Corner

From the bustling streets of Marrakesh to the lively markets of Lagos, street food in Africa is an experience that tantalizes all senses. Savor Ghanaian Kelewele, spicy, crisp fried plantains that tease and enchant the palate, or lose yourself in the comforting embrace of South African Bunny Chow, a hollowed loaf of bread brimming with spicy curry.

A Vegetarian's Paradise

In nations like Ethiopia, where fasting days (often vegetarian) are numerous, a splendid array of plant-based dishes enchant the palate. Injera, a sourdough flatbread, gracefully cradles a variety of vibrant, flavorful stews, presenting a feast that is as nutritious as it is flavorful.

Meat, Fire, and Celebration: The African Barbecue

Conversations around African cuisine cannot exclude the rich, smoky barbecue traditions. Picture the 'Nyama Choma' of East Africa, where gatherings and celebrations are punctuated with mounds of meticulously grilled, marinated meat, symbolizing unity, festivity, and shared joy.

26
MESOAMERICA AND THE FOODS OF THE NEW WORLD

Today, our taste buds invite us to traverse the vibrant and eclectic world of Mesoamerican cuisine, a realm where an illustrious past marries an innovatively vibrant present.

The Maize Labyrinth: Journeying Through the Core of Mesoamerican Diet

As we step into the corridors of Mesoamerican culinary history, the omnipresence of maize, or corn, is unmistakably evident. From the traditional Mexican tortillas to the Salvadoran pupusas, maize has been the backbone, both nutritionally and culturally, of Mesoamerican societies for millennia. Picture the ancient Mayans and Aztecs, cultivating their terrains with an astute understanding of the land, shaping a cuisine that still pulsates through the region today.

The Sacred Trilogy: Maize, Beans, and Squash

Dubbed the "Three Sisters" by Native American tribes, the triad of maize, beans, and squash not only governed the agricultural practices of the ancients but also epitomized a culinary doctrine that was both nutritious and sustainable. These three ingredients, intertwined in growth and in the plate, crafted meals that were a symbiotic symphony of flavors and health.

Chocolātl: The Divine Elixir

Ah, chocolate! That bewitching concoction that has enamoured palates globally was once the drink of the gods, utilized by ancient Mesoamericans not just as a beverage but as currency and offering. Picture frothy, rich, and sometimes spicy potions, far removed from the sweetened versions we know today, guiding your senses through ancient rituals and royal courts.

Chiles and Salsas: A Dance of Heat and Flavor

Engage your palate with the myriad of chiles - from the subtle to the scorching, crafting salsas and sauces that are artworks in their own right. Mesoamerican cuisine is a melody where chiles play the bold, vibrant notes, imparting depth, zest, and an unforgettable kick to the dishes they grace.

Tamales: Parcels of Culinary Heritage

Nestled in corn husks or banana leaves lie tamales, steamed parcels that echo the varied, multi-faceted aspects of Mesoamerican cuisine. Whether filled with spicy meats, sweet fruits, or rich, dark mole, tamales are edible narratives of the people, enveloping tales of daily life, festivals, and familial bonds.

Tacos: A Global Love Affair

Could we explore Mesoamerican cuisine without lingering over tacos? From the soft, homemade tortillas to the plethora of fillings, ranging from grilled meats and fish to regional cheeses and locally grown vegetables, tacos encapsulate the principle of simplicity, skill, and sincerity that governs the culinary traditions of the region.

From Past to Present: A Culinary Renaissance

In the contemporary world, chefs and home cooks alike are
resurrecting and reimagining ancient practices, blending the old
with the new, crafting a Mesoamerican culinary narrative that is as
rich, varied, and enchanting as the civilizations from which it
emerged.

27

THE MIDDLE EASTERN PALETTE: A TAPESTRY OF FLAVORS

It's the enchanting culinary domain of the Middle East, where every bite is an embrace, each aroma a cherished whisper of tales from ancient lands and enduring traditions.

A Symphony of Spices

Imagine strolling through a bustling souk, where the air is thick with the tantalizing aromas of spices – turmeric, sumac, za'atar, and saffron painting the atmosphere with their vibrant hues and captivating scents. The spices not only lend their colors and fragrances but also weave a tapestry that binds the myriad flavors of Middle Eastern cuisine into a harmonious melody that dances gracefully upon the palate.

Bread: The Quintessential Companion

From the soft, pillowy pita to the wafer-thin lavash, bread in the Middle East is not merely a staple; it's an inseparable companion to meals, a vessel that conveys flavors and textures, and a symbol of hospitality and community. It partakes in every feast, humble or lavish, absorbing the rich juices, and swaddling delicate morsels from mezze platters.

Mezze: A Feast of Diversity

Speaking of mezze, these delightful assortments of appetizers offer a kaleidoscopic view into the regional diversities and similarities within Middle Eastern cuisine. Hummus, tabbouleh, baba ganoush, and falafel often find their place amid an array of other local specialties, inviting people to linger, to savor, and to share.

Grains and Legumes: Sustenance and Simplicity

Venture with us through the fields of barley, wheat, and lentils, where age-old farming practices have nurtured civilizations. Dishes like mujaddara – a humble, comforting blend of rice, lentils, and caramelized onions – tell tales of sustenance and simplicity, revealing the essence of a cuisine that flourishes on balanced flavors and nutritious ingredients.

The Sacred Olive

Olive trees, with their gnarled trunks and silvery leaves, stand as sentinels of history and heritage in Middle Eastern landscapes. The olive, with its fruit and oil, permeates through the cuisine, imparting its subtle, earthy flavors and healthful blessings to dishes, while also symbolizing peace and prosperity.

Kebabs and Grills: The Communal Feast

Underneath the starlit skies, gatherings around grills and kebabs forge connections and celebrate togetherness. From the sumptuous shawarmas to the delicate koftas, the mastery of grilling meats in Middle Eastern cuisine is not just a culinary endeavor but a social affair that cements relationships and crafts memories.

Sweets: Honeyed Bites of Tradition

Embark on a sojourn into the sweet indulgences of baklava, ma'amoul, and halva, where layers of flaky pastry meet melanges of nuts and honey, forming luscious delights that are often synonymous with hospitality, festivity, and benevolence in the Middle East.

In each spice, every shared plate, and all gatherings around a hearty meal, Middle Eastern cuisine tells stories of civilizations, of trade routes and invasions, of traditions, and a timeless culture that honors hospitality, community, and the sheer joy of savoring good food.

28

ISLAND FOODS: NAVIGATING PACIFIC AND CARIBBEAN CULINARY SEAS

Join us as we embark on a savory adventure across the expansive Pacific and the vibrant Caribbean, exploring the flavors and stories etched into the rich tapestry of their respective cuisines.

Aloha, Pacific Flavors

Beginning our journey across the vast Pacific, we find ourselves amidst the lush terrains and crystal-clear waters of Hawaii. Here, the 'Aina (land) and Kai (sea) bestow their bounties generously upon the tables of locals. Poi, made from the taro plant, shares the plate with succulent pork in traditional Luaus, where food becomes a celebration of life, community, and harmony with nature.

Navigating further into the Pacific, we discover how the ocean's vastness incubates diversity. From the earthy, umami-rich flavors of fermented fish in the Philippines to the vibrant and fresh offerings of poke bowls in Polynesia, the Pacific intertwines the abundance of sea and land in a luscious culinary dance.

Caribbean: A Melodic Culinary Blend

As we sail into the warm, inviting waters of the Caribbean, our senses are greeted by a symphony of aromas and flavors, born from a rich history of exploration, colonization, and the confluence of diverse cultures. The indigenous, African, European, and Asian influences weave a culinary melody that is both vibrant and comforting.

Imagine a Jamaican jerk chicken, its skin kissed by the flames and imbued with a smoky, spicy marinate that sings of African influences and Taino techniques. Visualize, too, the creamy, hearty Callaloo, an indigenous stew of leafy greens, sometimes accentuated with coconut milk, crab, or salted meat, echoing the diverse voices of the Caribbean islands.

Rice, Spice, and Everything Nice

The story of island foods would be incomplete without highlighting the pivotal role of rice and spices. Rice, whether it's the sticky varieties preferred in the Pacific or the long-grained types adored in the Caribbean, forms the heart of many island meals, grounding the vibrant, spicy, and aromatic flavors with its subtle, comforting presence.

Spices tell tales of trade routes, of colonizers and slaves, of pain and resistance, and ultimately, of a beautiful melding of cultures and cuisines. From the pungent punch of pimento in the Caribbean to the zesty zing of ginger in the Pacific, spices navigate through every dish, narrating stories of times gone by and lands far away.

Sweet Notes from the Tropics

Let's not forget the sweet serenade of the tropical fruits, the mangoes, pineapples, guavas, and coconuts, that so generously lend their flavors to both savory and sweet dishes alike, creating a culinary repertoire that sings of sun-kissed soils and the nurturing warmth of island climates.

As we drift on the culinary seas from one island to another, we absorb not just the flavors and techniques but also the spirit of the islands – a spirit that revels in the abundance of land and sea, that celebrates community and togetherness, and that perpetuates a heritage rich with stories, struggles, and triumphs through every shared meal.

29

FUSION FOODS AND THE MELDING OF CULINARY CULTURES

Welcome to the intricate world of fusion foods, where we'll discover how disparate flavors, ingredients, and techniques from varying cultures weave together, forming new, exciting, and often surprising culinary tapestries.

Where the Culinary Streams Merge

Imagine an Italian pizza adorned with luscious pieces of sashimi-style fish, or a creamy Indian curry served encased in a delicate, flaky French pastry. Fusion food reflects a melting pot of cultural experiences, driven by the journeys, migrations, and imaginative experiments of people across the globe. It is, at its heart, a testament to our collective, intertwined histories and a celebration of our shared future.

The Interplay of Elements

Within the embrace of fusion cuisine, contrasting elements conspire, cavort, and commingle. There is the interplay of flavors, where sweet might meet savory, spicy might rendezvous with cool, and bitter might find an unexpected ally in sour. Textures, too, play a vital role—imagine the crunch of a crispy, fried element giving way to a tender, softly cooked morsel.

Challenging and Celebrating Traditions

This amalgamation is far more than simply mashing up dishes from different cultures—it's a craft that requires a delicate balance, an intimate knowledge of the ingredients, flavors, and techniques being fused, and a respectful nod to their origins and traditions. Fusion cuisine challenges chefs to step out of their comfort zones, to see beyond the traditional boundaries and envisage something startling yet familiar, innovative yet rooted in authenticity.

Celebrated Fusions and Unlikely Pairings

From the now-ubiquitous Tex-Mex, where spicy Mexican flavors are given a hearty Texan twist, to the innovative Korean Tacos of the Los Angeles food truck scene, the instances of successful fusion foods highlight how culinary creativity knows no bounds. Then there are examples like Japanese-Peruvian (Nikkei) cuisine, where umami-rich Japanese ingredients find a home amidst the bold, fresh flavors of Peru, or the Indo-Chinese cuisine, a beloved culinary genre in India that marries fiery Indian spices with classic Chinese cooking techniques.

The Journeys Behind the Flavors

Behind every fusion dish, there's a story – tales of migrants carrying their culinary heritage across oceans and borders, of explorers discovering new ingredients and flavors in distant lands, of chefs daring to experiment, innovate, and occasionally, court controversy. The Vietnamese Bánh Mì, for example, speaks of French colonial influence with its crisp baguette, yet is unequivocally Vietnamese with its vibrant, pickled vegetables, cilantro, and spicy, savory proteins.

Navigating the Fusion Future

In our contemporary globalized world, fusion foods continue to evolve, reflecting our interconnectedness and the dynamic, ever-changing nature of culinary culture. It not only survives but thrives by being fluid, adaptable, and endlessly inventive.

30

STREET FOODS AROUND THE WORLD

In this chapter, we'll saunter through the lively lanes of the world, nibbling on the heart and soul of many cultures: street food. Ah, street food, that marvelous concoction of flavors, wrapped in tradition and often, newspaper! It's where culinary arts meet the masses, where gourmet is not restricted by four walls and is free for all to savor.

An Unpretentious Culinary Maestro

While high-end restaurants often get lauded for their culinary innovations, street food, in its humble attire, has been quietly orchestrating a symphony of flavors without the accolade of shiny stars or reviews. The real essence of a culture's culinary expertise is often found not in refined restaurants, but on the bustling streets amongst common folk. It's a symphony where every bite tells a story, every spice sings a local tune, and every stall has a history intertwined with the community.

Where Every Bite Tells a Story

Imagine biting into a crispy, juicy 'Aloo Tikki' (potato cutlet) on the busy streets of Delhi, where the tang of tamarind chutney meets a spicy green coriander mint concoction. Or perhaps a steaming bowl of Vietnamese 'Pho' from a street-side stall in Hanoi, where fresh herbs meld effortlessly with rich, fragrant broth and tender slices of beef. Each offering is not merely a dish but a narrative of the people, their history, struggles, celebrations, and everyday life.

A Melting Pot of Flavors and Cultures

Across the vast expanse of the globe, street food morphs, adapts, and imbibes the local ethos. In Mexico, 'Tacos' are not just a quick bite but a reflection of the rich, diverse culinary landscape that varies from one region to the next. Whereas, in the tiny lanes of Bangkok, 'Pad Thai' whispers tales of culinary evolution, where Thai ingredients dance with flavors introduced by Chinese traders.

Vibrancy, Vitality, and a Touch of Rebellion

The world of street food is perpetually vibrant and vivacious. It's a world where recipes are not penned down but passed through generations, where measurements are not through cups or spoons but instinct, and where cooking is not a chore but a celebration. This is a domain where innovation thrives, where a vendor may choose to suddenly add a new ingredient, or try a different technique, not bounded by the strict rules that often govern formal cooking.

The Community Around Street Foods

Moreover, it is also a world where food becomes a tool for social interaction. Street food vendors do not just sell food; they become landmarks, meeting points, and even, unofficial community centers. And you, the eater, are not just a customer but a part of a larger, unspoken fraternity, bound by the love for flavors, and an appreciation for the uncelebrated maestros behind the carts.

Sustainability and Local Produce

Often sourcing local produce and ingredients, these street vendors also present a model of sustainability and support to local economies. They demonstrate that scrumptious meals don't always require exotic ingredients but can be whipped up with what's available, fresh, and in season.

A Culinary Walk Through Streets

Buckle up, dear reader, as we embark on this gastronomic journey through the vibrant streets of the world. There will be stops, detours, and perhaps a little indigestion, but oh, the stories we'll collect, and the flavors we'll discover, will indeed be treasures to cherish. From steaming dim sums in the crowded lanes of Hong Kong to the grilled kebabs of the Middle East, our journey will weave through continents, narrating tales of spices, textures, and, most importantly, the undying spirit of the common man and woman.

Savoring the Streets, Bite by Bite

As we meander through our culinary tour, let's not merely skim through the menagerie of flavors but rather dive deep, experiencing the nuance and history with each bite.

India: A Symphony of Spices

India, a vast subcontinent, offers an eclectic mix of street foods, each narrating a unique tale. Mumbai's 'Vada Pav', a spiced potato patty snuggled in a soft bun, talks of the city's bustling life and the need for quick, hearty meals. 'Pani Puri', tiny puffed balls filled with spicy tamarind water, whispers of timeless traditions and regional variations that morph as you traverse from north to south and east to west.

Thailand: A Dance of Sweet, Sour, and Spicy

The streets of Thailand are a kaleidoscope of flavors and aromas. With 'Pad Thai', rice noodles stir-fried with tofu or shrimp, peanuts, and bean sprouts, you experience a balance that is quintessentially Thai – sweet, sour, spicy, and salty, all in one bite. And then there's 'Mango Sticky Rice', a simple yet profound dessert, telling tales of Thailand's lush landscapes and bountiful harvests.

Italy: Savoring La Dolce Vita

In Italy, street food often echoes the warmth of its people and the richness of its lands. 'Arancini', deep-fried rice balls stuffed with a plethora of fillings like mozzarella, peas, or ragù, speaks of Sicily's vibrant culture and historical influences. Meanwhile, 'Gelato', though globally renowned, offers a chilled, decadent scoop of Italian indulgence, tradition, and meticulous craftsmanship.

Mexico: A Flavorful Fiesta

Navigating through Mexico, one encounters 'Tacos' in numerous avatars, each variant reflecting local preferences and ingredients. The 'Tlayudas' of Oaxaca, often dubbed as Mexican pizza, narrate stories of indigenous cultures and the amalgamation of flavors over centuries. And who can forget 'Churros', the sweet, crispy delights that have traversed borders and been embraced by various cultures worldwide!

Japan: Simplicity and Perfection

Japanese street food, while minimalistic, brings forth maximum flavor and texture. 'Takoyaki', octopus-filled dough balls, and 'Okonomiyaki', a savory pancake, offer a window into the Japanese ethos of balance, simplicity, and respect for ingredients. The unassuming 'Taiyaki', a fish-shaped cake typically filled with sweet red bean paste, embodies the Japanese knack for combining visual aesthetic with culinary skill.

Lebanon: A Medley of Fresh and Zesty

Lebanese street food is a testament to the country's knack for melding freshness with hearty flavors. 'Falafel', deep-fried chickpea balls, and 'Shawarma', slow-cooked, thinly sliced meat, both wrapped in a pita with an assortment of fresh veggies and tangy tahini, showcase the Middle Eastern penchant for combining robust and zesty flavors with fresh, crisp textures.

Vietnam: A Melange of Colonial and Native

Vietnam's street food scene carries whispers of its colonial past intermingled with robust indigenous culinary traditions. 'Bánh Mì', a baguette filled with a variety of ingredients such as meats, vegetables, and condiments, is a perfect exemplar of this fusion, marrying French influence with Vietnamese flair.

South Africa: A Culinary Ode to Diversity

In South Africa, 'Bunny Chow', a hollowed loaf of bread filled with curry, tells tales of Indian indentured laborers, adaptation, and the beautiful, complex culinary tapestry woven from myriad cultural threads.

Let's move forward on our journey, where every corner turned unveils a new aroma, a new flavor, and a new story. Street food is not just sustenance; it's a living, breathing aspect of a culture, an unspoken, yet profoundly articulate language of a people, and a tradition that effortlessly binds generations. With every step, we're not just spectators but active participants in a timeless, flavorful dialogue that spans the globe. So, let's keep wandering, tasting, and celebrating the boundless, spirited world of street food!

31
CULINARY CELEBRATIONS AND FESTIVALS GLOBALLY

Where merriment and culinary artistry meld, creating a palette where every hue is a flavor, and every flavor is a fragment of a culture's soul. In this chapter, we embark on a joyful journey, exploring the vivacious world of culinary celebrations and festivals that sprinkle our globe with a delightful mixture of tradition, innovation, and of course, splendid food.

Imagine: The air is dense with aromas, your footsteps synchronized with the rhythmic dance of revelry, and your taste buds tingling in anticipation of the culinary wonders ahead. Welcome to a world where every bite tells a story of heritage, every sip sings a song of camaraderie, and every dish is a timeless tradition dished out with love and gusto.

Spain: Tomatoes Tell a Tale

Our adventure begins in Buñol, Spain, amidst the uproarious mirth of "La Tomatina". Here, tomatoes are not just a fruit; they're amicable weapons in a jovial battle, and instruments of unity in diversity. Amidst the spirited tomato fights, the culinary scene blossoms with 'Paella' and tapas, embodying the Spanish spirit of community and shared joy over meals.

China: A Lunar Culinary Voyage

Whisking away to China, we witness the enthralling spectacle of the Lunar New Year, where food is not merely consumed but celebrated and revered. Dumplings ('Jiaozi') become parcels of prosperity, while rice cakes ('Nian Gao') symbolize growth and the promise of a better year. Every dish is imbued with symbolism, each bite a whisper of good fortune and communal bonds.

USA: A Grateful Harvest

Journeying to the USA, we're greeted by the warm, inviting aromas of Thanksgiving. Turkey, cranberries, and pumpkins are not mere ingredients but symbols of a grateful harvest. The meal is a homage to unity, a culinary canvas where indigenous and immigrant foodways weave a rich, diverse tapestry, echoing tales of unity, gratitude, and the amalgamation of myriad culinary journeys.

India: A Festival of Flavors

In India, we navigate through the vibrant chaos of Diwali, the festival of lights. Amidst the flickering lamps and sparkling fireworks, the air is redolent with the sweet perfume of 'Gulab Jamuns' and the spicy allure of savory snacks. The variety is astounding, each region contributing to an intricate culinary mosaic that tells tales of historical, regional, and familial traditions.

Germany: Beers and Cheers

Next, we find ourselves amidst the lively brouhaha of Oktoberfest in Germany. Amidst the clinking of beer mugs, the aroma of sausages and pretzels wafts through the air. Here, food and drink are not mere consumables but an embodiment of camaraderie, historical brewing excellence, and a shared love for hearty, comforting meals.

Ghana: Uplifting the Yam

In Ghana, we dance through the Homowo Festival, a vibrant celebration of yams. These earthy tubers are transformed into 'Kpekple', and amidst the lively beats and colorful processions, food becomes a connection to the earth, a symbol of abundance and a bountiful harvest, and an offering of gratitude.

Brazil: A Carnival of Culinary Joy

Who could forget Brazil, where Carnival transforms the streets into a pulsating sea of colors, rhythms, and flavors? Amidst the samba beats and dazzling costumes, the food is a fiesta of Afro-Brazilian and native influences, where 'Feijoada' and 'Acarajé' dance in a vibrant celebration of flavors, history, and the indomitable Brazilian spirit.

From the ceremonious to the boisterous, every festival, every culinary celebration around the world is a window into the heart of a culture. It's a shared table where traditional recipes, generational secrets, and innovative twists are passed around, savoring the essence of humanity's shared love for celebrations and food. Our journey through these culinary celebrations is a delightful reminder of the universal joy found in food, festivity, and the fervent spirit of togetherness.

32

THE FOOTPRINTS OF COLONIALISM ON CUISINES

The footprints of colonialism, subtle yet indelible, have meandered through the kitchens of the colonized, intertwining with native culinary traditions to create an intricate tapestry of flavors, techniques, and ingredients that have paved the paths of modern cuisines.

The Spices of India

Picture this: The sun dips below the horizon in the Indian subcontinent, casting long shadows over bustling spice markets. The British, Dutch, and Portuguese navigated treacherous seas, drawn by black pepper, cardamom, and a treasure trove of spices. While the colonizers left, the meshing of culinary worlds endured. Curries found a home in British dining, while Indian cuisine embraced potatoes and tomatoes, weaving them into the rich, spicy tapestry of its food story.

The Culinary Carousel of the Caribbean

Sailing toward the Caribbean, the amalgamation of indigenous, African, and European culinary techniques births a vibrant, soulful cuisine. The dark chapters of slavery and colonization cannot be undone, but amidst the sorrowful tales, a resilient, rich, and robust culinary tradition arose. Ackee and Saltfish, emblematic of Jamaican cuisine, tells a story of adaptation, creativity, and survival against the colonial backdrop.

The Flavors of Indo-Chinese Fusion

Consider the meeting of soy with curry, the harmonizing of wok-frying with aromatic spices. The British colonization of the Indian subcontinent and parts of Southeast Asia birthed a fascinating culinary subplot: Indo-Chinese cuisine. A zesty, savory, and spicy affair that took the robust flavors of India and waltzed them gracefully with the umami and sour notes prevalent in Chinese cuisine.

The Sweet (and Savory) Impact on African Cuisine

In the African continent, diverse culinary narratives absorbed, adjusted, and sometimes resisted colonial influences. Cassava, introduced by the Portuguese, embedded itself into African cuisines, while peanuts (groundnuts) from the New World became a crucial ingredient in West African stews and sauces. From the spicy peri-peri of Mozambique to the groundnut soups of Ghana, colonial footprints mingled with traditional practices, creating innovative and enduring culinary traditions.

A Sip of Indonesian Coffee

Glide to Indonesia, where the Dutch craving for exotic spices and resources left an indelible mark. Coffee, once a jealously guarded Arab secret, found new roots in the fertile Indonesian soil, forever intertwining with the nation's identity and economy. Rendang, now celebrated as a quintessential Indonesian dish, quietly whispers tales of trade, travel, and colonial enterprise through its layers of flavor.

The Vietnam-France Culinary Affair

Let's meander through the aromatic streets of Vietnam, where the French colonial legacy permeates through sips of coffee and bites of Banh Mi. The culinary exchange introduced baguettes, pâtés, and coffee to Vietnam, which were then embraced and transformed into uniquely Vietnamese creations, marrying local ingredients and French staples in a curious culinary dialogue.

Navigating through this complex, intertwined culinary landscape, we witness a captivating dance of resistance, adaptation, and innovation as colonized nations amalgamated foreign ingredients and culinary techniques with their own, crafting the diverse, rich food tapestries we celebrate today.

33

FOOD, IDENTITY, AND CULTURAL PRESERVATION

If you've ever found comfort in the warm, familiar aroma wafting from a pot of a traditional family dish, you've sensed that powerful connection between our culinary practices and our personal and collective identities.

Whispers of Ancestors in Every Bite

It all begins with a single bite. That first mouthful that transports us back through time, connecting us with our roots, our heritage, and the stories of our ancestors. Whether it's the complex layers of a hearty lasagna, the spicy kick of a traditional curry, or the comforting simplicity of a bowl of rice, every dish has a story to tell, a link to a past that is deeply intertwined with our cultural identity.

Safeguarding a Legacy with Ingredients and Techniques

Take a moment to imagine how culinary traditions, handed down through generations, become a tangible connection to our history, our heritage, and our ancestors. When we knead the dough as our grandmothers did, or when we utilize a particular spice blend that

has been in our culture for centuries, we are not merely cooking;
we are preserving and perpetuating a rich cultural legacy. From the
homemade pasta of Italy to the fermented kimchi of Korea, each
culinary practice safeguards a piece of history, a fragment of
identity.

The Resilience in Culinary Stories

Journeying from one region to the next, observe the culinary
tapestry that speaks volumes about the trials, tribulations, and
triumphs of the people. Consider the gumbo of Louisiana, a dish
born from a mingling of diverse cultures and scarce resources,
embodying innovation, survival, and a rich, collective identity.
Similarly, the "soul food" of the African American community
narrates stories of endurance, resistance, and resourcefulness,
providing sustenance for the body and the soul amidst adversities.

The Diplomacy of Dining Tables

As we further our exploration, notice how culinary diplomacy has
unfolded over the centuries, where food becomes a medium
through which nations communicate, relate, and negotiate. The
cross-pollination of culinary traditions, whether through trade,
migration, or conquest, often results in a delightful mosaic of
flavors, textures, and techniques that symbolize the blending of
cultures, mutual respect, and understanding.

Preservation through Celebration

Let's also revel in the joyous celebrations where food takes center
stage, becoming a symbol of unity, heritage, and cultural pride.
From the lantern-lit streets during the Mooncake Festival in China
to the vibrant, flavorful spectacle of India's Diwali, these festive
occasions transcend beyond mere celebrations, emerging as crucial
moments for cultural and culinary preservation.

As we meander through these tales, we'll explore how, in the face
of globalization and modernization, communities across the globe
are striving to preserve their culinary identities, safeguarding their

heritage, narrating their histories, and celebrating their cultures through the universal and timeless language of food.

The Imperative of Culinary Conservation

In a world that's rapidly changing, where globalization often propels a homogenized culinary culture, there's an urgency to conserve and cherish the diverse tapestry of culinary identities. Recipes whispered from elders, techniques honed through generations, and flavors passed down like heirlooms—all are under threat of being lost to time.

Educating and Empowering the Next Generation

Yet, there's hope in the form of dedicated individuals, communities, and organizations striving to protect their culinary heritage. They are the guardians of traditions, who teach the young and empower the community to keep these legacies alive. Cooking classes, oral histories, and community cookbooks become tools of education and empowerment, passing on culinary knowledge like a torch to the next generation.

Restaurants as Cultural Ambassadors

Restaurants, often referred to as ambassadors of culture, play a pivotal role in preserving and promoting culinary identities. Chefs, as modern-day torchbearers, celebrate the flavors of their heritage while introducing them to a wider audience. Dining at these establishments becomes a cultural exchange, where customers not only savor dishes but also absorb the stories, histories, and the essence of a culture.

Culinary Tourism: A Path to Preservation

Culinary tourism, a burgeoning trend, allows travelers to immerse themselves in the local food scene. In these journeys, tourists not only savor authentic flavors but also contribute to the preservation of culinary traditions by supporting local artisans, markets, and food festivals. In this way, the act of eating becomes a form of cultural conservation.

Resilience and Adaptation

Cultural preservation through food is not static; it's dynamic and adaptive. It allows for innovation while respecting tradition. It embraces change while safeguarding identity. Consider the evolution of sushi in Japan, which has embraced diverse ingredients and techniques while staying true to its essence, or the rise of modern Mexican cuisine, where ancient flavors are reimagined with contemporary finesse.

Conclusion: A Feast of Diversity

In the tapestry of global cuisines, every thread is precious, every dish a narrative, and every bite a celebration of the human spirit. As we navigate the intricacies of food, identity, and cultural preservation, we realize that the flavors on our plates are not just sustenance; they are windows into the rich, diverse world of cultures.

34

THE GLOBAL IMPACT OF AGRICULTURAL PRACTICES

As we dive deeper into the world of culinary cultures, it's essential to recognize that the roots of any cuisine lie in the earth itself. The agricultural practices of a region are like the quiet choreographers behind the culinary stage, shaping what grows on the land, what is harvested, and ultimately, what lands on our plates. In this chapter, we embark on a journey to explore how agricultural practices, both historical and contemporary, have left indelible marks on global cuisines.

The Terroir of Tradition

Imagine the rolling vineyards of France, where the very soil imparts character to the grapes. Or picture the terraced rice paddies of Southeast Asia, where centuries-old practices mold the very essence of the rice. Agricultural traditions rooted in the terroir—the unique combination of soil, climate, and culture—infuse ingredients with distinctive flavors and qualities that define regional cuisines.

Rice: The Lifeblood of Asia

Let's begin our exploration with rice, an agricultural staple that sustains billions in Asia. From the fragrant Basmati in India to the glutinous varieties in Japan, rice cultivation practices have sculpted Asian culinary traditions. The intricate rituals of planting, harvesting, and even the way rice is consumed reflect a profound connection between agriculture and cuisine.

Mediterranean Magic: Olive Groves and Vineyards

Heading west to the Mediterranean, olive groves and vineyards dot the landscape, embodying the deep-rooted agricultural practices of the region. The ancient Greeks celebrated olive oil for its culinary and medicinal virtues, while the Romans elevated the art of winemaking to new heights. These practices persist today, infusing Mediterranean cuisines with olive oil's golden richness and the nuanced flavors of regional wines.

The Maize of the Americas

In the Americas, the agricultural practices of indigenous cultures have played a pivotal role in shaping the culinary landscape. Corn, or maize, cultivated through centuries-old methods, is a linchpin of indigenous diets. From tortillas in Mexico to polenta in Italy, the global impact of maize is unmistakable, thanks to ancient cultivation techniques and reverence for this vital crop.

The Sea and Sustainable Practices

Not all agriculture happens on land. Sustainable fishing practices, passed down through generations, sustain coastal communities and influence cuisines worldwide. Think of the centuries-old techniques of Japanese fishermen, yielding delicate sushi and sashimi, or the art of Mediterranean fishermen, which provides fresh seafood for the iconic bouillabaisse.

Modern Agricultural Challenges

However, as we celebrate the rich tapestry of agricultural traditions, we must also confront modern challenges. Industrialization, monoculture farming, and environmental degradation have raised concerns about the sustainability of our food systems. Climate change threatens crop yields and disrupts traditional agricultural calendars, impacting the availability of key ingredients.

The Global Exchange of Ideas

In our interconnected world, agricultural practices and culinary traditions continue to cross borders. The exchange of ideas, ingredients, and techniques through trade, migration, and globalization has led to a fusion of flavors. As we'll explore in the upcoming chapters, this global exchange enriches our culinary experiences and broadens our palates.

Conclusion: The Plate and the Plow

Agricultural practices are the silent architects of our global culinary cultures, shaping what we eat and how we eat it. They are the foundation upon which culinary traditions are built. In this chapter, we've scratched the surface of a vast field of knowledge, one that touches every aspect of our culinary world.

35
A CULINARY TOUR OF INDIGENOUS TRIBES

Our culinary journey takes an exciting turn as we step into the vibrant, diverse world of indigenous tribes. These communities, often overlooked in mainstream narratives, are culinary treasure troves, offering an array of flavors, techniques, and traditions deeply rooted in their lands and cultures. Join us as we embark on a tour that celebrates the resilience and culinary richness of indigenous tribes across the globe.

The Wisdom of Traditional Knowledge

Indigenous communities have an intimate connection with the land and its resources. Passed down through generations, their traditional knowledge encompasses sustainable agricultural practices, wild foraging, and unique cooking techniques that harmonize with nature. In their world, food is not just sustenance; it's a sacred bond with the earth.

The Spirit of Sharing: Potlucks and Feasts

In North America, the Potlatch tradition of indigenous tribes is a testament to their generosity and communal spirit. These grand gatherings involve sharing food, stories, and cultural wealth, strengthening the bonds of the community. Salmon, a symbol of abundance, is often the centerpiece, prepared using ancestral techniques like smoking and drying.

Breadroot and Bison: Plains Indigenous Cuisine

Traveling to the Plains of North America, we encounter the culinary traditions of indigenous tribes like the Lakota and Dakota. Bison, revered as a source of life, is prepared in various forms, from roasted meat to pemmican, a mixture of dried bison meat and berries. Breadroot, a starchy root vegetable, offers sustenance and flavor, showcasing the Plains tribes' resourcefulness.

Amazon Rainforest: A Cornucopia of Flavors

Venturing to the Amazon rainforest, we find the culinary legacy of indigenous tribes like the Yanomami. Here, biodiversity is celebrated in every meal. Exotic fruits, tubers, and Amazonian fish are central to their diets. Cassava, transformed into various dishes like farofa and casabe, reflects their expertise in sustainable agriculture and preparation techniques.

Maori: Hāngi and Cultural Revival

In New Zealand, the Maori people have revived their traditional culinary practices, including the hāngi. This unique cooking method involves using heated stones buried in the earth to cook meat and vegetables, infusing them with smoky, earthy flavors. It's a beautiful example of how indigenous communities are preserving their culinary heritage and connecting with their roots.

Inuit and the Arctic Diet

As we journey north to the Arctic, we encounter the culinary traditions of the Inuit people. Their diet primarily consists of seafood, including seals, whales, and fish, expertly prepared to withstand the harsh climate. Fermented foods like muktuk (whale skin and blubber) offer essential nutrients and a unique taste of the Arctic.

Conclusion: A World of Flavorful Stories

In this chapter, we've merely scratched the surface of the rich culinary tapestry woven by indigenous tribes worldwide. Each tribe, with its distinct flavors and traditions, has a story to tell—a story of resilience, respect for nature, and a deep connection to the land.

SECTION III

The Modern Plate: Food, Fitness, and Well-being

36

UNPACKING MODERN DIET DILEMMAS

Welcome to Part III of our culinary journey, where we dive headfirst into the intricate relationship between food, fitness, and well-being in the modern age. Our journey thus far has taken us through ancestral wisdom, global culinary cultures, and the richness of indigenous traditions. Now, we step into the complex world of contemporary diets, where choices are abundant, information is overwhelming, and health is paramount.

The Modern Plate: A Multifaceted Dilemma

In our fast-paced, interconnected world, the modern plate reflects a kaleidoscope of choices and contradictions. On one hand, we have unprecedented access to diverse cuisines and ingredients from around the world, enriching our culinary experiences. On the other, we grapple with the challenges of health, sustainability, and ethical concerns that shape our food choices.

The Rise of Processed Foods

The modern diet dilemma is punctuated by the rise of processed foods, often laden with preservatives, added sugars, and unhealthy

127

fats. Convenience has become a driving force, but it comes at a price: the potential compromise of our health. As we'll explore, understanding the intricacies of food labels and making informed choices is crucial.

The Quest for Health and Nutrition

The pursuit of health and nutrition has given birth to a myriad of diets—Paleo, Keto, Vegan, Mediterranean, and more. Each touts its unique benefits, making it challenging for individuals to navigate the dietary landscape. We'll unpack these diets, shedding light on their principles and potential advantages.

Food as Medicine

In recent years, the concept of "food as medicine" has gained traction. From the anti-inflammatory properties of turmeric to the heart-healthy benefits of olive oil, we'll explore how certain foods offer therapeutic effects, and how incorporating them into our diets can promote well-being.

Sustainability and Ethical Eating

The modern plate is not just about nutrition; it's also about ethics and sustainability. We face the dilemma of balancing our dietary choices with environmental concerns, animal welfare, and fair labor practices. As conscientious consumers, we'll delve into the impact of our food choices on the planet and society.

The Mindful Plate

Amidst the complexities of the modern diet, mindfulness emerges as a guiding principle. Eating mindfully involves savoring each bite, being attuned to hunger and fullness cues, and making conscious choices that align with our health and values. We'll explore how mindfulness can reshape our relationship with food.

Conclusion: Navigating the Modern Plate

In this chapter and the ones to follow, we'll embark on a journey to unpack the modern diet dilemmas, seeking clarity amidst the chaos of choices. We'll explore the latest scientific research, dispel myths, and offer practical insights to help you make informed decisions about what goes on your plate.

As we navigate the modern plate together, remember that the path to well-being is not one-size-fits-all. It's a personalized journey that considers your unique preferences, cultural influences, and health goals. Join us in unraveling the complexities of the modern diet, making choices that nourish both body and soul, and finding a path to balance, health, and culinary satisfaction.

The Hidden Health Hazards of Processed Foods

Let's begin by addressing the elephant in the room: processed foods. While they offer convenience, they often come with a hidden cost to our health. Studies have linked the consumption of highly processed foods to an increased risk of obesity, heart disease, and diabetes. These products are typically high in added sugars, unhealthy trans fats, and sodium, while lacking essential nutrients.

Navigating Food Labels: A Key to Healthy Choices

Understanding food labels is crucial in making informed choices. Look out for red flags like excessive added sugars and unhealthy fats. A diet rich in fruits, vegetables, whole grains, lean proteins, and healthy fats is associated with lower risks of chronic diseases. The Mediterranean diet, for instance, has been extensively studied and is linked to improved heart health, longevity, and cognitive function.

Balancing Macronutrients: The Role of Carbs, Fats, and Proteins

The macronutrient balance in our diets plays a significant role in our health. Carbohydrates, often viewed with skepticism, are an essential source of energy. However, not all carbs are created equal. Whole grains, vegetables, and fruits offer valuable nutrients and fiber, while refined carbohydrates can lead to blood sugar spikes. Healthy fats, such as those found in olive oil, nuts, and fatty fish, are associated with a reduced risk of heart disease. Proteins, whether from animal or plant sources, are crucial for muscle repair and overall well-being.

Dietary Diversity: The Key to Micronutrients

Micronutrients, including vitamins and minerals, are essential for various bodily functions. A diverse diet that includes a rainbow of fruits and vegetables ensures we get a wide array of these micronutrients. For example, vitamin C from citrus fruits boosts our immune system, while calcium from dairy or fortified plant-based sources supports bone health.

Food as Medicine: A Scientific Perspective

The idea of "food as medicine" isn't just a catchy phrase; there's solid scientific backing. Certain foods are rich in bioactive compounds with therapeutic properties. Turmeric, for instance, contains curcumin, known for its anti-inflammatory effects. Omega-3 fatty acids in fatty fish like salmon have been linked to reduced risk of heart disease. These dietary choices can be powerful tools in maintaining health and preventing disease.

Sustainable Eating: A Global Imperative

The sustainability of our food choices has far-reaching implications for the planet. Studies show that adopting plant-based diets and reducing meat consumption can significantly reduce greenhouse gas emissions. Sustainable farming practices, such as organic farming and regenerative agriculture, promote healthier ecosystems. As consumers, we can make a difference by choosing sustainably sourced foods and reducing food waste.

Mindful Eating: A Holistic Approach to Well-being

In the midst of nutritional complexities, mindfulness emerges as a valuable ally. Mindful eating involves savoring each bite, paying attention to hunger and fullness cues, and fostering a positive relationship with food. Research indicates that practicing mindfulness while eating can lead to healthier eating habits, improved digestion, and reduced emotional eating.

37
THE PROCESSED FOOD PHENOMENON

In this chapter, we'll uncover the multifaceted world of processed foods, examining their impact on our diets, health, and the global food landscape.

The Rise of Processed Foods

Processed foods have become an integral part of modern diets. These products, often convenient and shelf-stable, have gained popularity due to their extended shelf life and ease of consumption. From breakfast cereals to frozen dinners, they cater to our fast-paced lifestyles.

The Hidden Culprits: Added Sugars and Unhealthy Fats

One of the major concerns associated with processed foods is their high content of added sugars and unhealthy fats. These ingredients are often used to enhance flavor and palatability. However, excessive consumption of added sugars, especially in sugary beverages and snacks, is linked to obesity, type 2 diabetes, and heart disease. Trans fats, commonly found in processed snacks and baked goods, can raise bad cholesterol levels and increase the risk of heart disease.

Sodium Overload: The Salt Trap

Another issue with processed foods is their high sodium content. While salt is a necessary nutrient, excessive sodium intake is a known risk factor for hypertension and heart disease. Processed foods, particularly canned soups, snacks, and processed meats, can contribute significantly to our daily sodium intake.

The Fiber Gap: Processing Removes Nutrients

Processing often removes essential nutrients and dietary fiber. Whole grains are stripped of their bran and germ layers, reducing their fiber and nutrient content. This can lead to a lack of satiety and potential overconsumption, as fiber-rich foods help control appetite.

The Complex World of Food Labels

Understanding food labels is a critical skill in navigating the processed food landscape. Terms like "low-fat," "natural," and "organic" can be misleading. It's essential to scrutinize ingredient lists for added sugars, unhealthy fats, and high sodium levels. Choosing products with shorter ingredient lists and recognizable ingredients is a wise strategy.

Beyond Nutrition: The Environmental Impact

The processed food phenomenon isn't just a health concern; it also has far-reaching environmental implications. The production and packaging of processed foods contribute to greenhouse gas emissions and plastic waste. Adopting sustainable eating habits that prioritize whole, minimally processed foods can help mitigate these environmental issues.

A Balanced Approach

While it's crucial to be mindful of the potential pitfalls of processed foods, a balanced approach to diet is key. Not all processed foods are harmful; some provide convenience without sacrificing nutrition. Frozen fruits and vegetables, for example, can be nutritious choices. The key is to choose wisely, prioritize whole, fresh foods, and limit the consumption of heavily processed options.

Conclusion: Navigating the Processed Food Maze

In this chapter, we've ventured into the complex world of processed foods, unearthing their impact on our health and the environment. While they offer convenience, processed foods often come with hidden health risks. By understanding food labels, being aware of added sugars and unhealthy fats, and choosing whole, minimally processed options, we can make informed dietary choices.

38

DIETARY GUIDELINES: A HISTORICAL PERSPECTIVE

In our ongoing journey through the complexities of the modern plate, it's crucial to understand how dietary guidelines have evolved over time. These guidelines, shaped by scientific research and societal needs, play a pivotal role in shaping our eating habits, health outcomes, and the food industry itself.

The Early Years: Basic Nutrition Principles

The concept of dietary guidelines emerged in the early 20th century when nutritional scientists began studying the link between diet and health. The first dietary guidelines focused on essential nutrients like vitamins and minerals. During World War II, guidelines aimed to ensure proper nutrition for soldiers and civilians in times of rationing.

The Birth of Food Groups: The Four Food Groups Era

In the mid-20th century, dietary guidelines took a new form with the introduction of food groups. The "Four Food Groups" model categorized foods into milk, meat, fruits and vegetables, and grains.

This approach simplified dietary recommendations and aimed to ensure a balanced intake of essential nutrients.

The Revolution of Dietary Fat: The Low-Fat Era

By the 1970s, concerns about heart disease led to a shift in dietary recommendations. The low-fat era emerged, with guidelines advocating for reduced fat consumption, particularly saturated fats found in animal products. This led to the proliferation of low-fat and fat-free products in the market.

A Changing Landscape: The Mediterranean Diet and Cultural Influences

In recent decades, dietary guidelines have evolved to embrace cultural diversity and regional diets. The Mediterranean diet, characterized by abundant fruits, vegetables, whole grains, and healthy fats, gained recognition for its heart-healthy benefits. This shift acknowledged that a one-size-fits-all approach might not be suitable for diverse populations.

The Complex Modern Plate: Balancing Macronutrients

Today's dietary guidelines emphasize a balanced intake of macronutrients—carbohydrates, fats, and proteins. They recognize the importance of whole grains, lean proteins, healthy fats, and a variety of fruits and vegetables. These guidelines aim to empower individuals to make informed choices that align with their health goals.

The Role of Science and Industry

Scientific research continues to shape dietary guidelines. Advances in nutritional science provide insights into the role of specific nutrients and dietary patterns in preventing chronic diseases. However, the influence of the food industry cannot be ignored. Food companies often shape public perceptions through marketing and lobbying efforts.

The Future of Dietary Guidance: Personalization and Sustainability

The future of dietary guidelines is likely to focus on personalization and sustainability. Advances in genetics and nutrition science may enable personalized dietary recommendations tailored to an individual's genetic makeup and health status. Additionally, sustainability considerations, such as the environmental impact of food choices, are gaining importance in dietary guidance.

Conclusion: A Continuously Evolving Plate

In this chapter, we've journeyed through the historical evolution of dietary guidelines. These guidelines have played a significant role in shaping our understanding of nutrition, health, and food choices. As we navigate the complexities of the modern plate, it's essential to remain aware of the historical context and the dynamic nature of dietary guidance. By staying informed and making choices that align with our individual needs and values, we can navigate the modern plate with confidence and well-being.

39

FITNESS THROUGH THE AGES

As we delve deeper into the realm of the modern plate, we must not overlook the vital companion to nutrition: fitness. Our understanding of fitness has evolved significantly over time, reflecting changes in our lifestyles, societal norms, and scientific knowledge. In this chapter, we'll embark on a journey through the history of fitness to explore how it has shaped our approach to well-being.

The Ancient Pursuit of Physical Excellence

The concept of physical fitness can be traced back to ancient civilizations such as Greece, where the Olympic Games celebrated athleticism and strength. Greek philosophers like Hippocrates emphasized the importance of exercise for health. In China, practices like Tai Chi and martial arts date back thousands of years, promoting balance and physical harmony.

The Industrial Revolution and the Emergence of Gym Culture

The Industrial Revolution brought about significant changes in our way of life. As people moved from agrarian communities to urban centers, physical activity decreased. This shift prompted the emergence of gym culture in the 19th century, with the belief that exercise could counter the sedentary effects of industrialization.

The Fitness Renaissance: Aerobics and Home Workouts

The mid-20th century saw a resurgence of interest in fitness, driven by figures like Jack LaLanne and Jane Fonda. Aerobic exercise became a household term, and home workouts gained popularity with the advent of fitness videos. The focus shifted from pure athleticism to overall health and wellness.

Science Meets Fitness: The Role of Research

Scientific research in the 20th century began to unravel the complexities of exercise physiology and its impact on health. Studies showed the benefits of regular physical activity in reducing the risk of chronic diseases such as heart disease, diabetes, and obesity. This knowledge reinforced the importance of fitness in our lives.

The Digital Age: Technology and Fitness Tracking

The 21st century ushered in a new era of fitness, intertwined with technology. Wearable fitness trackers and smartphone apps revolutionized the way we monitor and engage with our physical activity. These tools allow individuals to set goals, track progress, and gain insights into their health.

Fitness Trends: From CrossFit to Mind-Body Practices

Fitness trends have diversified to cater to various preferences and goals. CrossFit emphasizes functional, high-intensity workouts, while yoga and mindfulness practices promote mental and physical balance. Group fitness classes, boutique studios, and online platforms offer a range of options to suit individual needs.

The Holistic Approach: Nutrition and Fitness Synergy

Today, our understanding of well-being emphasizes the synergy between nutrition and fitness. Proper nourishment provides the fuel for physical activity, while exercise supports overall health and complements dietary choices. This holistic approach underscores the importance of balance in our modern lives.

Conclusion: A Lifelong Journey

The history of fitness is a testament to our enduring pursuit of well-being. From ancient cultures to the digital age, the importance of physical activity remains steadfast. As we navigate the complexities of the modern plate, let us remember that fitness is not a destination but a lifelong journey. By embracing the wisdom of the ages and harnessing the tools of the present, we can cultivate a life marked by vitality, health, and a profound connection between nutrition and fitness.

40
METABOLISM: ANCIENT BODIES IN A MODERN WORLD

In our exploration of the modern plate and its impact on our well-being, we come face to face with the intricate and ancient concept of metabolism. This fundamental physiological process is a cornerstone of our existence, yet it faces unique challenges in the context of the modern world.

The Ancient Engine of Life

Metabolism, in simple terms, is the complex set of chemical reactions that sustain life. It's the process by which our bodies convert food into energy, building blocks for tissues, and substances needed to support vital functions. This remarkable process has been at the core of human existence for millennia.

Metabolism in the Ancestral Context

In ancient times, our ancestors relied on metabolism to transform the foods they hunted and foraged into energy for survival. The efficiency of their metabolic systems was honed by evolution to maximize energy extraction from scarce resources, making efficient use of every calorie.

The Modern Plate: A Metabolic Challenge

Fast forward to the modern world, where the plate is laden with an abundance of highly processed, calorie-dense foods. Our ancient metabolic systems, finely tuned for scarcity, now grapple with an unprecedented surplus of calories. This dietary transition has contributed to the global rise in obesity and related health issues.

Metabolism and Weight Regulation

Metabolism plays a crucial role in weight regulation. Basal metabolic rate (BMR), the energy expended at rest, varies among individuals. Genetics, age, muscle mass, and lifestyle factors all influence BMR. A slower BMR can make it challenging to maintain or lose weight, especially in the modern environment.

Metabolism and Nutrient Processing

Metabolism also governs how our bodies process macronutrients —carbohydrates, fats, and proteins. The modern diet's emphasis on refined carbohydrates and unhealthy fats can disrupt metabolic balance, leading to insulin resistance and metabolic syndrome.

Adaptations for the Modern Plate

While our metabolic systems are ancient, they possess remarkable adaptability. Incorporating whole, unprocessed foods, regular physical activity, and balanced meals can support a healthy metabolism. These practices align with our ancestral dietary patterns, promoting efficient energy use and overall well-being.

The Role of Physical Activity

Physical activity is a potent modulator of metabolism. Exercise increases muscle mass, which, in turn, boosts BMR. It also enhances insulin sensitivity, helping the body regulate blood sugar more effectively. Regular physical activity is a cornerstone of metabolic health in the modern world.

Metabolism in the Ancestral Context

To truly grasp the significance of metabolism in the modern world, it's essential to look back at our ancestral context. Our ancient forebears led lives deeply intertwined with the rhythm of nature, where food was scarce, and energy conservation was paramount.

Survival in a World of Scarcity

In the ancestral world, food wasn't as readily available as it is today. Hunter-gatherer societies relied on foraging for plant-based foods and hunting for animal protein. The irregularity of successful hunts and seasonal variations in the availability of fruits and vegetables meant that our ancestors often faced periods of food scarcity.

Metabolic Adaptations for Survival

In response to these challenges, our bodies evolved metabolic adaptations designed to extract the maximum energy from the limited food sources available. When food was scarce, our metabolic rate could decrease to conserve energy. This adaptive feature allowed our ancestors to survive periods of famine and make the most of every calorie consumed.

Efficiency in Energy Utilization

Additionally, the ancestral metabolic system was highly efficient at converting consumed nutrients into energy. Fat storage was prioritized, enabling individuals to store energy for lean times. This mechanism, essential for survival in a feast-and-famine environment, becomes a double-edged sword in the modern era of constant abundance.

The Modern Plate: A Clash of Timelines

Fast forward to the present, and we find ourselves in a world of dietary abundance and sedentary lifestyles. The modern plate, laden with processed foods rich in refined sugars and unhealthy fats, presents a stark contrast to the ancestral diet. Our metabolic systems, finely tuned for scarcity, now grapple with an overabundance of calories and a different nutritional landscape.

Conclusion: A Tale of Two Worlds

Understanding metabolism in the ancestral context highlights the incongruity between our ancient bodies and the modern plate. The adaptations that once ensured our survival now pose challenges in an environment of calorie excess. To navigate this clash of timelines, we must harness our knowledge of metabolism, embrace a diet closer to our ancestral roots, and stay active—a trifecta that supports our ancient engines in the modern world.

41
GUT HEALTH: PROBIOTICS, FERMENTED FOODS, AND MICROBIOME

We turn our attention to an area of growing importance: gut health. The intricate ecosystem of our digestive system, including the gut microbiome, plays a vital role in our overall health and deserves a closer look.

The Gut: More Than a Digestive Organ

While we often associate the gut with digestion, it's a dynamic and complex system with a multitude of functions. It's not just a processing plant for food; it's a hub for communication between our bodies and trillions of microorganisms that reside within.

The Microbiome: A World Within Us

At the heart of gut health is the microbiome—a vast community of bacteria, viruses, fungi, and other microorganisms that call our digestive system home. These microscopic inhabitants are not passive passengers; they actively participate in digestion, immune function, and even influence our mood and behavior.

Probiotics: The Friendly Allies

Probiotics are beneficial bacteria that we can introduce into our gut to bolster its health. These microorganisms, often found in fermented foods like yogurt, kefir, and sauerkraut, help maintain a balanced gut microbiome. Probiotics have been associated with improved digestion, enhanced immune function, and even mood regulation.

Fermented Foods: Culinary Alchemy

Fermented foods have been part of human diets for centuries. Through the process of fermentation, natural microbes transform raw ingredients into a treasure trove of flavors and health benefits. Examples include kimchi, kombucha, and miso. These foods not only provide probiotics but also enhance the digestibility and nutritional value of the ingredients.

The Gut-Brain Connection: Mood and More

Recent research has uncovered the intriguing gut-brain connection. The gut communicates with the brain through a network known as the gut-brain axis. Emerging evidence suggests that the composition of the gut microbiome can influence mood, stress levels, and even cognitive function. A balanced gut microbiome appears to be crucial for mental well-being.

Nourishing Your Microbiome: Fiber and Diversity

To support a healthy gut microbiome, it's essential to feed it well. Fiber-rich foods like whole grains, fruits, and vegetables provide nourishment for beneficial gut bacteria. A diverse diet, one that includes a wide array of foods, promotes microbial diversity, which is associated with better health outcomes.

The Modern Plate and Gut Health

The modern plate can be a double-edged sword for gut health. Highly processed foods, low in fiber and laden with artificial additives, can disrupt the delicate balance of the gut microbiome. On the other hand, a diet rich in whole, unprocessed foods and fermented delicacies can be a boon for gut health.

Conclusion: Cultivating Gut Wellness

In this chapter, we've dived into the intricate world of gut health, exploring the microbiome, probiotics, fermented foods, and the gut-brain connection. Nurturing your gut is a journey towards overall well-being. By embracing a diet that supports microbial diversity and incorporating probiotic-rich foods, you can cultivate a balanced gut ecosystem that contributes to your health and vitality in the modern world.

42

WEIGHT MANAGEMENT: ANCIENT WISDOM, MODERN STRATEGIES

In our exploration of the modern plate and its implications for well-being, one of the most prevalent and pressing concerns is weight management. Striking a healthy balance between nutrition, physical activity, and lifestyle is essential for maintaining a healthy weight. In this chapter, we'll explore how ancient wisdom and modern strategies converge to address this timeless challenge.

The Ancient Wisdom of Balance

Our ancestors, guided by necessity and nature, possessed an inherent understanding of balance when it came to food and activity. They didn't have the conveniences and abundance of the modern world, so their diets were often characterized by whole, unprocessed foods. Their active lifestyles were driven by the need to hunt, gather, and perform physical tasks.

The Modern Plate: A Landscape of Choices

Fast forward to today, and our plates are filled with choices beyond what our ancestors could have imagined. Processed foods, high in sugar and unhealthy fats, are readily available, while physical activity has become optional rather than essential. The modern plate can lead to weight-related challenges.

Calories In vs. Calories Out: A Timeless Equation

Weight management often boils down to a fundamental equation: calories in vs. calories out. Consuming more calories than our bodies need leads to weight gain, while a calorie deficit results in weight loss. While this concept remains constant, modern food choices and sedentary lifestyles have made it more challenging to strike a balance.

The Role of Macronutrients

Beyond calorie quantity, the quality of our calories matters. The macronutrients—carbohydrates, fats, and proteins—play distinct roles in hunger regulation and metabolism. A balanced intake of these nutrients, aligned with our ancestral dietary patterns, can support weight management.

Mindful Eating: An Ancient Practice in a Modern World

Mindful eating, rooted in ancient practices, encourages us to savor each bite, listen to our body's hunger and fullness cues, and cultivate a mindful relationship with food. This approach can help us navigate the modern plate with awareness and moderation.

Physical Activity: Modern Challenges, Timeless Benefits

Physical activity remains a cornerstone of weight management. In our modern, technology-driven world, we often lead sedentary lives. However, incorporating regular movement, whether through structured exercise or daily activities, is essential for calorie expenditure and overall health.

The Power of Support and Education

Seeking support and education are vital components of successful weight management. Access to reliable information, guidance from healthcare professionals, and social support networks can empower individuals to make informed choices and stay committed to their goals.

The Role of Psychological Well-being

While the science of weight management often focuses on physical factors, it's crucial not to overlook the psychological aspects. Stress, emotional eating, and mental well-being are integral components of the weight management equation.

Ancient practices such as yoga and meditation, which prioritize mental and emotional balance, can provide valuable tools for addressing stress and emotional eating. These practices help individuals cultivate a healthier relationship with food and their bodies.

Nutrient Density: A Key to Satiety

Another concept that bridges ancient wisdom with modern strategies is nutrient density. Ancient diets were inherently nutrient-dense, with whole, unprocessed foods providing an abundance of vitamins, minerals, and dietary fiber. These nutrient-rich foods promote satiety and can help regulate calorie intake.

In the modern world, focusing on nutrient-dense choices—such as colorful vegetables, lean proteins, and whole grains—can enhance the feeling of fullness and satisfaction, making it easier to manage calorie consumption.

Cultural Perspectives on Eating

Our cultural heritage often shapes our relationship with food. Ancient cultural practices, like communal meals and rituals, can offer valuable insights into mindful eating and portion control. By honoring these traditions, individuals can embrace a balanced approach to food that extends beyond mere nutrition.

The Quest for Sustainable Habits

Sustainability is an emerging consideration in the realm of weight management. Ancient cultures often had a deep respect for the environment and its resources. By adopting sustainable eating habits that prioritize local, seasonal, and minimally processed foods, individuals can contribute to both their own well-being and the health of the planet.

Conclusion: A Holistic Approach

In this chapter, we've ventured deeper into the multifaceted world of weight management. While the principles of calories in vs. calories out remain at its core, it's clear that a holistic approach is essential. By blending ancient wisdom with modern strategies, individuals can navigate the complexities of the modern plate with mindfulness, balance, and a deep understanding of the interplay between nutrition, physical activity, and mental well-being. In doing so, they can strive for not just weight management but overall health and vitality.

43

NUTRITIONAL DEFICIENCIES AND THE MODERN DIET

As we continue our journey through the modern plate and its impact on well-being, one of the persistent concerns is the potential for nutritional deficiencies. Despite the abundance of food choices in today's world, many individuals are not getting the essential nutrients their bodies need. In this chapter, we'll explore the reasons behind nutritional deficiencies in the modern diet and their consequences.

The Paradox of Plenty

At first glance, it might seem counterintuitive that nutritional deficiencies persist in a world of plenty. However, the modern diet is characterized by both overconsumption of certain foods and underconsumption of critical nutrients. Here are some factors contributing to this paradox:

Highly Processed Foods: The modern plate often includes an abundance of highly processed foods that are calorie-dense but nutrient-poor. These foods are often stripped of essential vitamins, minerals, and fiber during processing.

Excessive Caloric Intake: Many people in the modern world consume excess calories, leading to weight gain. Paradoxically, this can occur alongside inadequate intake of essential nutrients. Individuals may fill up on calorie-laden, nutrient-poor foods while missing out on essential vitamins and minerals.

Food Choices: The modern diet tends to prioritize convenience and taste over nutritional content. Fast food, sugary beverages, and snacks high in unhealthy fats and sugars are readily available and often preferred over healthier options.

The Consequences of Nutritional Deficiencies

Nutritional deficiencies can have far-reaching consequences for health and well-being. Here are some common deficiencies and their potential effects:

Vitamin D Deficiency: Insufficient vitamin D can lead to weakened bones, increased risk of fractures, and even mood disorders.

Iron Deficiency: Iron is essential for transporting oxygen in the blood. Iron deficiency can result in anemia, fatigue, and decreased immune function.

Vitamin B12 Deficiency: This deficiency can cause fatigue, weakness, and neurological problems. It's especially common among vegetarians and vegans who don't consume animal products.

Calcium Deficiency: Inadequate calcium intake can weaken bones and increase the risk of osteoporosis.

Folate Deficiency: Folate is crucial for DNA synthesis and repair. A deficiency can lead to anemia and contribute to birth defects during pregnancy.

Addressing Nutritional Deficiencies

Addressing nutritional deficiencies involves making deliberate choices about the foods we consume. Here are some strategies:

Balanced Diet: Emphasize a balanced diet rich in whole, unprocessed foods. Fruits, vegetables, whole grains, lean proteins, and healthy fats provide a spectrum of essential nutrients.

Supplementation: In cases where dietary intake alone is insufficient, supplementation may be necessary. Consultation with a healthcare professional can guide appropriate supplementation.

Mindful Eating: Practicing mindful eating can help individuals become more aware of their food choices and portion sizes, promoting a more nutrient-rich diet.

Education and Awareness: Increasing awareness of the importance of balanced nutrition and its impact on health is crucial. Education can empower individuals to make informed dietary choices.

Conclusion: Nourishing the Body and Mind

In this chapter, we've explored the issue of nutritional deficiencies in the modern diet. While we live in an era of unprecedented food availability, it's vital to remember that the quality of our food choices matters just as much as quantity. By prioritizing whole, nutrient-dense foods and making informed dietary decisions, individuals can nourish not only their bodies but also their overall well-being.

44

THE SCIENCE BEHIND CRAVINGS AND ADDICTIONS

In our exploration of the modern plate and its impact on well-being, we can't overlook a powerful force that often influences our food choices: cravings and addictions. The allure of certain foods and the struggle to resist them are challenges many individuals face. In this chapter, we'll delve into the science behind cravings and food addictions to better understand their roots and consequences.

Cravings vs. Addictions: What's the Difference?

Before we dive into the science, it's important to distinguish between cravings and addictions. Cravings are strong desires for specific foods, often driven by taste preferences, memories, or emotional factors. Cravings can be a normal part of the human experience and are not inherently problematic.

Addictions, on the other hand, involve a loss of control over the consumption of a substance, in this case, certain foods. Food addiction shares similarities with substance addictions, such as drug or alcohol dependence. It's characterized by compulsive eating, cravings that are difficult to resist, and negative consequences for physical and mental health.

The Brain's Reward System

Cravings and addictions both have roots in the brain's reward system. When we consume foods that are pleasurable or high in sugar, fat, or salt, the brain releases neurotransmitters like dopamine, which create a sensation of pleasure and reinforce the desire to eat these foods.

Over time, repeated consumption of highly rewarding foods can lead to changes in the brain's reward pathways. The brain becomes more sensitive to these foods, making cravings more intense and difficult to resist. This phenomenon is similar to the way addictive substances affect the brain.

The Role of Emotional and Environmental Factors

Cravings and food addictions can also be influenced by emotional and environmental factors. Stress, boredom, and negative emotions can trigger cravings for comfort foods, which are often high in sugar and fat. Environmental cues, like the sight or smell of certain foods, can also trigger cravings.

The Modern Plate and Food Addictions

The modern plate can exacerbate the challenge of food addictions. Highly processed foods are designed to be hyper-palatable, often containing a combination of sugar, fat, and salt that stimulates the brain's reward system. These foods can be particularly difficult for individuals with food addictions to resist.

Consequences of Food Addictions

Food addictions can have serious consequences for physical and mental health. They can lead to overeating, weight gain, and the development of chronic conditions like obesity and type 2 diabetes. Food addictions can also take a toll on emotional well-being, leading to guilt, shame, and a negative cycle of emotional eating.

Addressing Cravings and Food Addictions

Addressing cravings and food addictions often requires a multi-faceted approach:

Awareness: Recognizing the triggers and patterns of cravings is the first step in managing them.

Mindfulness: Mindful eating techniques can help individuals become more aware of their food choices and break the cycle of emotional or addictive eating.

Support: Seeking support from healthcare professionals, therapists, or support groups can be invaluable for individuals struggling with food addictions.

Balanced Diet: A balanced diet that includes a variety of nutrient-dense foods can help stabilize blood sugar levels and reduce the intensity of cravings.

Conclusion: Navigating the Modern Food Landscape

In this chapter, we've explored the science behind cravings and food addictions. Understanding the neural and psychological processes at play can provide insight into the challenges individuals face in making healthy food choices. By combining awareness, mindfulness, and support with a balanced diet, individuals can navigate the modern food landscape and work towards healthier relationships with food.

45
SUGAR: A SWEET AND BITTER HISTORY

Sugar—its sweetness has captivated our taste buds for centuries, and its presence on the modern plate is ubiquitous. However, beyond its delightful taste lies a complex history and a growing concern about its impact on health. In this chapter, we'll explore the journey of sugar from a prized rarity to a dietary staple and delve into the bittersweet aspects of this ubiquitous ingredient.

The Sweetness of Sugar: A Historical Perspective

Sugar's history is as rich and complex as its flavor. It was first cultivated in ancient India and used as a medicinal substance before its culinary potential was realized. Sugar's journey from India to Persia, and eventually to Europe, made it a highly prized commodity during the Middle Ages.

Sugar and the Age of Exploration

The Age of Exploration in the 15th and 16th centuries marked a turning point for sugar. European powers established sugar plantations in colonies, such as the Caribbean and the Americas, leading to the mass production of sugar. This shift from rarity to abundance had far-reaching consequences.

The Bitter Legacy of the Sugar Trade

The sugar trade was fueled by the forced labor of enslaved people, leading to immense human suffering and exploitation. The transatlantic slave trade, driven in part by the demand for sugar, remains a dark chapter in history.

Ancient Origins of Sweetness

Sugar has ancient roots that stretch back thousands of years. Its early history can be traced to Southeast Asia, where sugarcane was first cultivated. The sweet juice extracted from sugarcane became a prized commodity in the region.

The Sugar Trade and Colonialism

As human societies evolved, so did the sugar trade. Sugarcane cultivation spread to the Middle East and eventually to the Mediterranean. In the medieval period, sugar was a luxury reserved for the wealthy. The demand for sugar played a significant role in the age of exploration and the colonization of the Americas, where sugar plantations became a lucrative industry.

The Industrial Revolution and Sugar Production

The Industrial Revolution brought about significant changes in sugar production. Advances in technology, such as steam engines and mechanized mills, made sugar more affordable and accessible to the masses. The rise of the sugar beet industry in Europe further expanded the availability of sugar.

The Modern Plate: Sugar's Ubiquity

Today, sugar is everywhere in our modern diet. It's not just found in sweets and desserts but also hidden in a multitude of processed foods, from condiments to packaged snacks. The average person consumes far more sugar than our ancestors could have imagined.

The Sweet Conundrum: Health Impact

While sugar adds delightful sweetness to our foods, its excessive consumption has raised concerns about its impact on health. High sugar intake has been linked to a range of health issues, including obesity, type 2 diabetes, and heart disease. It can also contribute to dental problems and sugar addiction.

Balancing Sweetness: Modern Challenges

Balancing our love for sweetness with the need for health is one of the challenges of the modern plate. Refined sugars, commonly used in processed foods, provide empty calories devoid of nutrients. They can lead to blood sugar spikes and crashes, exacerbating cravings and affecting energy levels.

Navigating the Sugar Landscape

To navigate the sweet and bitter history of sugar on the modern plate, individuals can:

- **Read Labels:** Check food labels for hidden sugars, often listed under various names like sucrose, high fructose corn syrup, and dextrose.

- **Choose Natural Sweeteners:** Opt for natural sweeteners like honey, maple syrup, or stevia, which can add sweetness with fewer refined sugars.

- **Limit Processed Foods:** Reduce the consumption of heavily processed foods and focus on whole, unprocessed options.

- **Practice Moderation:** Enjoy sweet treats in moderation, savoring them as occasional indulgences rather than daily staples.

Conclusion: A Sweet and Informed Choice

Sugar's journey from a rare luxury to a ubiquitous ingredient on the modern plate reflects the evolution of human tastes and desires.

While it continues to sweeten our lives, it's essential to approach sugar with awareness and moderation, making informed choices that prioritize both pleasure and health.

46
POPULAR DIETS: AN ANALYTICAL REVIEW

In the quest for optimal health and well-being, diets have played a significant role throughout history. Today, the landscape of popular diets is diverse and often bewildering. In this chapter, we'll take a closer look at some of the most prominent diets that have captured the attention of the modern plate and critically analyze their principles and impact.

1. Paleo Diet

The paleo diet, inspired by the eating habits of our ancient ancestors, emphasizes whole, unprocessed foods like lean meats, fish, fruits, vegetables, nuts, and seeds. It excludes grains, dairy, legumes, and processed foods.

Pros: The paleo diet encourages whole foods and minimizes processed ones, which can lead to improved nutrient intake and weight management.

Cons: Eliminating entire food groups can make it challenging to meet essential nutrient requirements. The diet's historical accuracy is also debated.

2. Mediterranean Diet

Based on the traditional diets of Mediterranean countries, this diet emphasizes fruits, vegetables, whole grains, legumes, nuts, and olive oil. It includes moderate amounts of fish, poultry, and dairy, with limited red meat consumption.

Pros: The Mediterranean diet is associated with numerous health benefits, including reduced risk of heart disease and improved longevity.

Cons: Some individuals may find it challenging to adopt due to cultural differences and preferences.

3. Ketogenic Diet

The ketogenic diet is a high-fat, low-carbohydrate eating plan designed to induce ketosis—a metabolic state where the body uses fat for energy instead of carbohydrates. It's used for weight loss and managing conditions like epilepsy.

Pros: The keto diet can lead to rapid weight loss and improved blood sugar control for some individuals.

Cons: It's a restrictive diet that may lead to nutrient deficiencies, constipation, and other side effects. Long-term health effects are still under study.

4. Vegan Diet

A vegan diet excludes all animal products, including meat, dairy, eggs, and even honey. It's based on plant-based foods like fruits, vegetables, grains, legumes, nuts, and seeds.

Pros: A well-balanced vegan diet can provide numerous health benefits, including reduced risk of heart disease and certain cancers.

Cons: Careful planning is required to ensure adequate intake of essential nutrients like vitamin B12, iron, and calcium. It may also require lifestyle adjustments.

5. Intermittent Fasting

Intermittent fasting involves cycling between periods of eating and fasting. Popular methods include the 16/8 method (fasting for 16 hours and eating within an 8-hour window) and the 5:2 diet (eating normally for 5 days and restricting calorie intake for 2 days).

Pros: Some studies suggest that intermittent fasting can aid in weight loss, improve insulin sensitivity, and support cellular repair.

Cons: It may not be suitable for everyone, and overeating during eating windows can negate its benefits. Long-term effects are still being researched.

6. Low-Carb Diet

Low-carb diets restrict carbohydrate intake, often focusing on protein and fat. They aim to control blood sugar levels and promote weight loss.

Pros: Low-carb diets can be effective for weight loss and may help control blood sugar in individuals with diabetes.

Cons: Restricting carbohydrates can limit fiber intake and increase the risk of nutrient deficiencies. It may also be challenging to sustain in the long term.

7. DASH Diet

The Dietary Approaches to Stop Hypertension (DASH) diet is designed to lower blood pressure. It emphasizes fruits, vegetables, whole grains, lean proteins, and low-fat dairy while limiting sodium intake.

Pros: The DASH diet is effective for reducing blood pressure and has a balanced approach to nutrition.

Cons: It may require careful planning to meet nutrient needs, and some individuals may find it difficult to adhere to the low sodium recommendations.

Conclusion: Personalization and Balance

The effectiveness of any diet depends on individual factors, including health goals, preferences, and lifestyle. Rather than adhering strictly to one diet, it's often beneficial to take a balanced approach, incorporating elements from various diets that align with your health objectives. Always consult with a healthcare professional or registered dietitian before making significant dietary changes to ensure they are appropriate for your unique needs and circumstances.

47

FOOD ETHICS AND SUSTAINABILITY

As we explore the modern plate and its impact on well-being, it's crucial to consider the ethical and sustainability dimensions of our food choices. In this chapter, we'll delve into the complex and interconnected issues surrounding the ethics of food production and the imperative of sustainability.

The Ethical Dilemmas of Food Production

Modern food production is fraught with ethical challenges that touch on a range of concerns:

- **Animal Welfare:** The treatment of animals in industrial farming has raised significant ethical questions. Crowded and inhumane conditions, routine use of antibiotics, and practices like debeaking in poultry farming have drawn criticism.

- **Environmental Impact:** The environmental consequences of large-scale agriculture, including deforestation, habitat destruction, and excessive water use, have ethical implications. These practices contribute to climate change and threaten biodiversity.

- **Food Waste:** The vast amount of food wasted at various stages of the supply chain, from production to consumption, raises ethical concerns in a world where hunger coexists with abundance.

- **Social Justice:** Disparities in access to nutritious food and fair treatment of workers within the food system highlight issues of social justice and food equity.

Sustainability: A Global Imperative

Sustainability in food production involves practices that meet current needs without compromising the ability of future generations to meet their own needs. It encompasses several key aspects:

- **Environmental Sustainability:** This involves minimizing the negative impact of agriculture on the planet by using resources efficiently, reducing greenhouse gas emissions, and protecting ecosystems.

- **Social Sustainability:** Social sustainability in food production considers the well-being of farm workers, fair labor practices, and the promotion of equitable access to food.

- **Economic Sustainability:** Sustainable agriculture aims to support the livelihoods of farmers and ensure economic viability for the long term.

The Modern Plate and Sustainable Choices

In the modern world, individuals have the power to make choices that align with food ethics and sustainability:

- **Supporting Local Agriculture:** Buying locally grown and produced foods supports small-scale farmers and reduces the carbon footprint associated with long-distance transportation.

- **Reducing Meat Consumption:** Choosing plant-based meals or reducing meat consumption can lessen the environmental impact of food production.

- **Minimizing Food Waste:** Avoiding food waste by planning meals, using leftovers, and supporting initiatives to redirect surplus food to those in need reduces the strain on resources.

- **Advocacy and Education:** Supporting and advocating for ethical food production practices and policies can drive positive change.

Conclusion: A Plate of Conscious Choices

The modern plate is not just about what we eat but also how our food choices impact the world around us. By considering the ethical implications of food production and embracing sustainability, individuals can transform their plates into symbols of conscious choices that prioritize the health of the planet, animal welfare, and social justice. In doing so, we contribute to a more sustainable and equitable food system for all.

48

VEGANISM AND PLANT-BASED DIETS: A MODERN ADOPTION?

Veganism and plant-based diets have gained significant attention in recent years, prompting many to wonder whether this shift towards more plant-centric eating is a modern phenomenon. In this chapter, we'll explore the roots of veganism and plant-based diets, their rise in the modern world, and their impact on health and sustainability.

The Historical Roots of Plant-Based Diets

The idea of abstaining from animal products for ethical, religious, or health reasons has ancient origins:

- **Ancient Religions:** Vegetarianism has been practiced by various religious groups, including Jainism, Buddhism, and certain sects of Hinduism, for centuries. These traditions often emphasize non-violence and compassion towards all living beings.

- **Philosophical Movements:** In the West, philosophical movements in ancient Greece and Rome explored the ethical aspects of abstaining from animal consumption.

- **Health Advocacy:** Historical figures like Pythagoras promoted plant-based diets for health reasons.

The Modern Resurgence

While plant-based eating has ancient roots, the modern resurgence of veganism and plant-based diets is closely tied to contemporary concerns:

- **Ethical Considerations:** The ethical treatment of animals has become a central focus of modern veganism. Documentaries and advocacy efforts have shed light on the treatment of animals in industrial farming, sparking widespread concern.

- **Health and Nutrition:** Research highlighting the potential health benefits of plant-based diets, such as reduced risk of heart disease, diabetes, and certain cancers, has contributed to their popularity.

- **Environmental Concerns:** Increased awareness of the environmental impact of meat production and its contribution to climate change has driven many to adopt plant-based diets as a sustainable choice.

The Modern Plate: A Shift Towards Plant-Centric Eating

The modern plate reflects a notable shift towards plant-centric eating:

- **Plant-Based Proteins:** Plant-based proteins, such as tofu, tempeh, legumes, and meat substitutes, have become increasingly accessible and appealing to a broader audience.

- **Plant-Forward Restaurants:** The rise of plant-based and vegan restaurants and menu options in mainstream eateries signifies a shift in consumer preferences.

- **Plant-Based Convenience Foods:** Supermarkets now offer a wide array of plant-based convenience foods, from dairy-free ice cream to meatless burgers, making it easier for individuals to adopt plant-based diets.

Health Considerations

Plant-based diets can offer numerous health benefits, such as lower cholesterol levels, improved weight management, and reduced risk of chronic diseases. However, individuals need to plan their diets carefully to ensure they receive all essential nutrients, including vitamin B12, iron, and calcium.

Sustainability Impact

One of the driving forces behind the adoption of plant-based diets is their lower environmental footprint. Producing plant-based foods typically requires fewer resources and generates fewer greenhouse gas emissions compared to animal agriculture.

Conclusion: A Modern Evolution

While the roots of plant-based diets extend deep into history, their resurgence in the modern world is marked by a convergence of ethical, health, and environmental concerns. As more people adopt plant-based diets and incorporate plant-centric choices into their meals, they participate in a global movement towards a more compassionate, sustainable, and health-conscious approach to eating.

49

HEALING FOODS AND HOME REMEDIES

Throughout history, humans have turned to the healing properties of food and home remedies to address a wide range of ailments and promote well-being. In this chapter, we'll explore the age-old tradition of using food as medicine and how it continues to shape the modern plate.

The Wisdom of Ancient Healing Foods

Across cultures, ancient traditions have recognized the healing potential of specific foods:

- **Herbs and Spices:** Culinary herbs and spices like ginger, turmeric, garlic, and mint have been used for their medicinal properties. They contain compounds with anti-inflammatory, antibacterial, and antioxidant effects.

- **Fermented Foods:** Fermented foods like yogurt, kefir, and kimchi contain probiotics that support gut health, digestion, and immunity.

- **Bone Broth:** Bone broth, made by simmering animal bones and connective tissues, is rich in collagen, amino acids, and minerals. It's believed to support joint health and improve skin.

- **Honey:** Honey, prized for its antibacterial properties, has been used as a natural remedy for coughs and sore throats.

Modern Science Meets Ancient Wisdom

Modern scientific research has validated many of these traditional beliefs:

- **Turmeric and Curcumin:** Curcumin, a compound in turmeric, has been studied for its anti-inflammatory and antioxidant properties, which may benefit conditions like arthritis.

- **Probiotics:** Scientific studies have confirmed the role of probiotics in supporting digestive health and even influencing mental well-being.

- **Fiber and Gut Health:** High-fiber foods like fruits, vegetables, and whole grains promote a healthy gut microbiome, with implications for overall health.

- **Omega-3 Fatty Acids:** Omega-3s found in fatty fish, flaxseeds, and walnuts have anti-inflammatory effects that may benefit heart and brain health.

Home Remedies in the Modern Kitchen

While the modern plate is filled with a diverse array of foods from around the world, the tradition of using food as medicine endures:

- **Ginger Tea:** A soothing remedy for nausea and digestive discomfort, ginger tea is a popular home remedy.

- **Chicken Soup:** Beyond its comforting properties, chicken soup has been shown to have anti-inflammatory effects and may help alleviate cold symptoms.

- **Garlic and Honey:** A mixture of garlic and honey is a folk remedy believed to boost the immune system.

- **Elderberry Syrup:** Elderberries are rich in antioxidants and are often used as a natural remedy for colds and flu.

Balancing Tradition and Science

While healing foods and home remedies have a valuable place in promoting well-being, it's essential to approach them with a balanced perspective:

- **Consultation:** Serious health concerns should be addressed with the guidance of healthcare professionals.

- **Integration:** Traditional remedies can complement modern medical treatments, but they should not replace them.

- **Individualized Approach:** What works for one person may not work for another, so it's crucial to listen to your body and adapt remedies to your needs.

Incorporating healing foods and home remedies into your modern plate can be a holistic approach to health and well-being. Let's explore more examples of these practices:

1. Herbal Teas: Herbal teas like chamomile, peppermint, and echinacea have been cherished for their therapeutic effects. Chamomile, known for its calming properties, is often used to promote relaxation and better sleep. Peppermint tea can aid digestion and alleviate headaches, while echinacea is believed to boost the immune system.

2. Apple Cider Vinegar: Apple cider vinegar has gained popularity as a home remedy for various ailments, including digestive issues and weight management. It's often diluted with water and consumed before meals.

3. Lemon Water: Starting the day with a glass of warm lemon water is a ritual for many. Lemons are rich in vitamin C and antioxidants, which may support immune health and hydration.

4. Turmeric Lattes: Turmeric lattes, also known as "golden milk," combine the anti-inflammatory properties of turmeric with the soothing effects of milk (or dairy-free alternatives) and a touch of sweetness. This beverage is touted for its potential to reduce inflammation and improve joint health.

5. Aloe Vera: Aloe vera, known for its skin-soothing properties, is sometimes consumed as a juice or added to smoothies. It's believed to support digestive health and may have anti-inflammatory effects.

6. Oatmeal Baths: Oatmeal baths are a soothing remedy for itchy or irritated skin. Ground oats can be added to warm bathwater to relieve discomfort caused by conditions like eczema.

7. Honey and Cinnamon: A mixture of honey and cinnamon is a popular home remedy believed to have diverse health benefits. It's claimed to help with issues ranging from colds and allergies to digestive problems and skin conditions. However, scientific evidence supporting these claims is limited.

8. Hot Water with Honey and Lemon: This classic home remedy is often used to soothe a sore throat and alleviate cold symptoms.

The warmth of the water, combined with the antibacterial properties of honey and the vitamin C in lemon, can provide relief.

Remembering the Holistic Approach

While these healing foods and home remedies can be valuable tools for supporting health, it's essential to approach them with a holistic mindset. They work best when integrated into a lifestyle that includes a balanced diet, regular exercise, adequate sleep, and stress management.

Additionally, individual responses to these remedies can vary. What brings relief to one person may not have the same effect on another. If you have chronic health concerns or are considering significant dietary changes, it's advisable to consult with a healthcare professional for personalized guidance.

Conclusion: The Healing Plate

In a world filled with pharmaceuticals and medical interventions, the healing power of food and home remedies remains a cherished and effective approach to well-being. By blending the wisdom of ancient traditions with modern scientific understanding, individuals can cultivate a "healing plate" that supports their health and vitality.

50
FITNESS REGIMENS AND DIETARY ADAPTATIONS

In the pursuit of optimal health and well-being, the relationship between diet and exercise is undeniable. This chapter delves into the symbiotic connection between fitness regimens and dietary adaptations, highlighting the importance of balancing both for a thriving, modern lifestyle.

Fueling Your Fitness

Whether you're a dedicated athlete or someone striving for a healthier lifestyle, the role of nutrition in your fitness journey is paramount:

- **Pre-Workout Fuel:** Eating a balanced meal or snack before exercise provides your body with the energy it needs to perform optimally. Carbohydrates, protein, and healthy fats are all part of the pre-workout equation.

- **Post-Workout Recovery:** After exercise, your body requires nourishment to repair muscles and replenish glycogen stores. Protein-rich foods, along with carbohydrates, are essential for recovery.

- **Hydration:** Staying adequately hydrated is critical for maintaining performance and preventing dehydration-related issues during workouts.

- **Micronutrients:** Vitamins and minerals play a vital role in overall health and can impact exercise performance. For example, calcium and vitamin D are essential for bone health, crucial for athletes.

Dietary Adaptations for Different Goals

Dietary adaptations are often tailored to specific fitness goals:

- **Muscle Gain:** Individuals aiming to build muscle typically increase their protein intake. They also focus on a well-rounded diet to support overall health and recovery.

- **Weight Loss:** Those seeking weight loss may focus on calorie control while still prioritizing nutrient-dense foods to meet their dietary needs.

- **Endurance Training:** Athletes engaging in endurance sports require a balance of carbohydrates to sustain energy levels during prolonged activity.

- **Flexibility and Balance:** Some fitness practices, like yoga and Pilates, prioritize flexibility and balance. While nutrition remains important, these disciplines may have more forgiving dietary requirements.

Diet Trends and Fitness Culture

The modern fitness landscape is influenced by diet trends, which can sometimes be polarizing:

- **High-Protein Diets:** Many fitness enthusiasts adopt high-protein diets to support muscle growth and recovery. However, it's essential to balance protein intake with other nutrients.

- **Keto and Low-Carb Diets:** Some athletes experiment with ketogenic or low-carb diets, believing they can enhance endurance and fat burning. These diets require careful planning to ensure adequate energy for workouts.

- **Plant-Based Diets:** Plant-based athletes are on the rise, demonstrating that plant-centric diets can provide the necessary nutrients for performance. Careful attention to protein sources is key.

- **Intermittent Fasting:** Intermittent fasting has gained popularity in fitness circles. Some claim it improves fat loss and muscle definition, but its suitability varies among individuals.

Finding Your Balance

The key to success in fitness and nutrition is finding the right balance that suits your goals and lifestyle. Here are some guiding principles:

- **Individualization:** What works for one person may not work for another. Tailor your diet to your specific goals and needs.

- **Consistency:** Consistency is essential in both diet and exercise. Long-term habits are more sustainable and effective.

- **Professional Guidance:** If you have specific fitness goals or dietary restrictions, consider consulting with a registered dietitian or fitness expert for personalized guidance.

- **Holistic Well-Being:** Remember that well-being is more than just physical fitness. Mental health, sleep, and stress management are crucial components of a healthy lifestyle.

Conclusion: A Harmonious Partnership

In the modern plate, diet and fitness are not separate entities but rather interconnected aspects of well-being. By approaching your fitness regimen and dietary choices with intention and balance, you can foster a harmonious partnership that supports your goals, whether they involve athletic performance, weight management, or simply living a healthier, more vibrant life.

51

MENTAL HEALTH: THE MIND-FOOD CONNECTION

While we often think about food and fitness in terms of physical health, it's crucial not to overlook their profound impact on mental well-being. In this chapter, we'll explore the intricate connection between what we eat and our mental health, shedding light on how our modern plate can nurture not only our bodies but also our minds.

The Gut-Brain Axis

One of the most fascinating revelations of recent research is the gut-brain axis—the bidirectional communication system between our gut and brain. The foods we consume have a direct influence on our gut microbiota, which, in turn, can affect our mental health:

- **Probiotics and Mood:** Probiotic-rich foods like yogurt and kefir contain beneficial bacteria that may positively impact mood and reduce symptoms of anxiety and depression.

- **Fiber and Mental Health:** A diet high in fiber supports a diverse gut microbiome, which has been associated with better mental health outcomes.

- **Inflammatory Foods:** Highly processed and inflammatory foods may contribute to chronic inflammation, which has been linked to mood disorders.

- **Nutrient Deficiencies:** Inadequate intake of essential nutrients like omega-3 fatty acids, B vitamins, and vitamin D can negatively impact brain function and mental health.

Eating for Emotional Well-Being

It's common for people to turn to comfort foods during times of stress or emotional distress. While occasional indulgence is part of a balanced approach to eating, it's essential to be mindful of your choices:

- **Stress Eating:** Emotional eating can lead to overconsumption of unhealthy foods, which may provide short-term comfort but can exacerbate emotional distress in the long run.

- **Mindful Eating:** Practicing mindful eating involves paying attention to your body's hunger and fullness cues, savoring each bite, and choosing foods that nourish both your body and mind.

- **Nutrient-Dense Choices:** Foods rich in antioxidants, such as fruits and vegetables, can help combat oxidative stress in the brain, potentially supporting mental clarity and emotional balance.

The Role of Omega-3 Fatty Acids

Omega-3 fatty acids, found in fatty fish like salmon, flaxseeds, and walnuts, are renowned for their heart-healthy benefits. However, they also play a crucial role in brain health:

- **Brain Structure:** Omega-3s are integral to the structure of brain cell membranes, influencing communication between brain cells.

- **Neurotransmitter Function:** These fatty acids can impact the production and function of neurotransmitters, which play a role in mood regulation.

- **Anti-Inflammatory Properties:** Omega-3s possess anti-inflammatory effects that may help reduce the risk of mood disorders.

Mindful Eating Practices

To harness the mind-food connection for improved mental health, consider adopting mindful eating practices:

- **Balanced Diet:** Consume a well-balanced diet rich in whole foods, including fruits, vegetables, whole grains, lean proteins, and healthy fats.

- **Probiotic Foods:** Incorporate probiotic-rich foods like yogurt, kefir, sauerkraut, and kimchi into your diet to support gut health.

- **Omega-3 Sources:** Include sources of omega-3 fatty acids in your meals, such as fatty fish, flaxseeds, and chia seeds.

- **Moderation:** Enjoy indulgent foods in moderation and be mindful of emotional eating triggers.

- **Professional Guidance:** If you're struggling with mental health issues, seek the guidance of a mental health professional or registered dietitian who can provide personalized recommendations.

Case Study - The Mediterranean Diet and Mental Health

Let's delve into a real-world case study to illustrate the profound impact of diet on mental health. Consider the Mediterranean diet, a dietary pattern renowned for its potential to support both physical and mental well-being.

The Mediterranean Diet: A Nutrient-Rich Approach

The Mediterranean diet is characterized by:

- Abundant fruits and vegetables

- Whole grains

- Healthy fats, particularly olive oil

- Moderate consumption of lean protein, mainly fish and poultry

- Limited red meat

- Occasional red wine in moderation

- Nuts, seeds, and legumes

Mental Health Benefits: The PREDIMED Study

The PREDIMED (PREvención con DIeta MEDiterránea) study, conducted in Spain, shed light on the relationship between the Mediterranean diet and mental health. This extensive study involved over 7,000 participants aged 55 to 80 and found:

- **Depression Risk Reduction:** Individuals who adhered closely to the Mediterranean diet were at a significantly lower risk of developing depression.

- **Improved Cognitive Function:** Participants following the diet exhibited better cognitive function over time, suggesting a potential protective effect against cognitive decline.

- **Reduced Inflammation:** The diet's anti-inflammatory components, such as omega-3 fatty acids and antioxidants, may contribute to improved mental health.

The Mind-Food Connection in Practice

This case study highlights how dietary patterns, such as the Mediterranean diet, can have a tangible impact on mental health. By emphasizing nutrient-rich foods and supporting a healthy gut microbiome, this approach contributes to emotional well-being.

Harnessing the Mind-Food Connection

As you explore your own journey of mental well-being through your modern plate, consider adopting the following strategies:

- **Experiment with Nutrient-Dense Foods:** Incorporate more fruits, vegetables, whole grains, and healthy fats into your meals.

- **Mindful Eating:** Pay attention to how different foods make you feel emotionally and physically, and adjust your choices accordingly.

- **Consult Professionals:** If you're managing mental health concerns, seek guidance from mental health professionals and registered dietitians to develop a personalized approach.

- **Celebrate Balance:** Remember that mental well-being is a holistic endeavor, and no single meal or dietary choice defines your emotional health. A balanced approach that includes physical activity, stress management, and supportive relationships is essential.

Conclusion: Nurturing Mind and Body

The modern plate is a powerful tool for nurturing not only your physical health but also your mental well-being. By making mindful food choices that support gut health, reduce inflammation, and provide essential nutrients, you can harness the mind-food connection to cultivate a state of balance and emotional resilience in your daily life.

52

BUILDING A BRIDGE: INTEGRATING ANCESTRAL DIET IN MODERN LIFE

In our quest for optimal health and well-being, the wisdom of our ancestors can serve as a guiding light. Building a bridge between ancestral diets and modern life means embracing the best of both worlds to create a sustainable and nourishing approach to eating.

The Ancestral Diet: A Glimpse into the Past

Ancestral diets, rooted in tradition and shaped by the availability of local foods, vary widely across cultures. Yet, they share common principles that align with our innate human biology:

- **Whole Foods:** Ancestral diets predominantly consist of whole, minimally processed foods like fruits, vegetables, lean proteins, and unrefined grains.

- **Seasonal Eating:** Traditional diets often revolve around seasonal foods, harnessing their natural flavors and nutritional benefits.

- **Balanced Nutrients:** These diets naturally strike a balance of macronutrients (carbohydrates, proteins, and fats) and are rich in essential vitamins and minerals.

- **Cultural Significance:** Food in ancestral diets isn't just sustenance; it carries cultural and social significance, fostering a sense of community and identity.

The Modern Plate: Challenges and Opportunities

Modern life brings both conveniences and challenges to our relationship with food:

- **Processed Foods:** Convenience foods, often highly processed and laden with additives, have become ubiquitous, contributing to health concerns.

- **Fast-Paced Lifestyles:** Busy schedules and the demand for quick meals can lead to less mindful eating.

- **Globalization:** Access to a wide variety of foods from around the world has expanded our culinary horizons but can sometimes lead to a disconnect from local and seasonal options.

Integrating Ancestral Wisdom: Practical Steps

Building a bridge between ancestral wisdom and modern life is an ongoing journey:

- **Embrace Whole Foods:** Prioritize whole, unprocessed foods in your diet. These foods provide essential nutrients and minimize exposure to artificial additives.

- **Mindful Eating:** Cultivate mindful eating practices, savoring each bite, and appreciating the sensory experience of food.

- **Local and Seasonal:** Whenever possible, choose local and seasonal produce. This supports local agriculture, reduces environmental impact, and provides fresher, more flavorful foods.

- **Cultural Heritage:** Explore your cultural heritage through food. Learn traditional recipes and cooking techniques that connect you with your roots.

- **Balanced Meals:** Strive for balanced meals that include a variety of foods and nutrients, reflecting the principles of ancestral diets.

The Flexibility of Ancestral Wisdom

Ancestral diets offer valuable guidelines, but they can be adapted to suit modern preferences and needs:

- **Plant-Centric Choices:** Emphasize plant-based foods while incorporating lean proteins, following the Mediterranean diet, for example.

- **Personalization:** Recognize that individual dietary needs vary. Tailor your approach based on your unique health goals, cultural background, and ethical beliefs.

- **Culinary Creativity:** Embrace the art of cooking and experiment with traditional and modern ingredients to create delicious and nutritious meals.

Case Study - The Blue Zones

To illustrate the integration of ancestral diet wisdom in modern life, let's explore a real-world case study: the Blue Zones. These are regions around the world where people live exceptionally long, healthy lives. Researchers have identified several common lifestyle factors in these areas, including diet.

Blue Zones and Diet: Key Insights

- **Okinawa, Japan:** In Okinawa, residents adhere to a traditional diet rich in vegetables, tofu, and small amounts of fish and lean meat. They consume fewer calories than the average Western diet and practice the principle of "Hara Hachi Bu," which means eating until they are 80% full.

- **Sardinia, Italy:** The Sardinian diet includes whole grains, beans, vegetables, and locally produced cheese and wine. It's characterized by simplicity and reliance on locally sourced, unprocessed foods.

- **Nicoya Peninsula, Costa Rica:** The traditional diet of Nicoyans centers on corn, beans, and squash. This trio of foods, known as "the three sisters," provides a balanced nutritional profile.

- **Ikaria, Greece:** Ikarians consume a Mediterranean-style diet that includes olive oil, vegetables, whole grains, and a moderate amount of goat's milk and wine. Wild greens and herbs are also staples.

Case Study Takeaways

The Blue Zones offer valuable insights into how ancestral dietary principles can be integrated into modern life:

- **Plant-Centric Eating:** These communities prioritize plant-based foods, which aligns with modern recommendations for health and sustainability.

- **Portion Control:** The practice of mindful eating and portion control supports overall health and longevity.

- **Local and Seasonal:** Blue Zones residents often rely on local and seasonal foods, reducing their ecological footprint and promoting fresh, nutrient-dense options.

Bringing It Home: Your Modern Plate

Drawing inspiration from the Blue Zones and other ancestral dietary wisdom, consider how you can integrate these principles into your modern plate:

- **Local Ingredients:** Explore locally grown and seasonal produce at farmers' markets and local food cooperatives.

- **Mindful Eating:** Embrace the concept of "Hara Hachi Bu" by listening to your body's hunger and fullness cues, and avoid overeating.

- **Balanced Choices:** Prioritize plant-based foods while incorporating lean proteins and healthy fats into your diet.

- **Culinary Exploration:** Experiment with traditional recipes and cooking techniques from your own heritage or other cultures to broaden your culinary horizons.

- **Community and Connection:** Share meals with loved ones, strengthening social bonds and enhancing the enjoyment of food.

Conclusion: A Harmonious Blend

Integrating ancestral diet wisdom into modern life is not about rigidly adhering to the past but rather finding a harmonious blend that nourishes both body and soul. By drawing inspiration from the culinary traditions of our ancestors while embracing the convenience and diversity of the modern plate, we can create a sustainable and fulfilling approach to food that supports our well-being for generations to come.

53

CASE STUDIES: SUCCESSFUL APPLICATION OF ANCESTRAL DIETS

In this chapter, we'll delve into real-world case studies that showcase the successful application of ancestral diets in modern settings. These stories illustrate how individuals and communities have harnessed the wisdom of their ancestors to achieve improved health and well-being.

Case Study 1: Mediterranean Diet for Heart Health

Meet Maria, a 60-year-old woman living in the United States.

Background: Maria had a family history of heart disease and was concerned about her own heart health. She decided to adopt the Mediterranean diet, inspired by her Greek heritage.

Application: Maria began incorporating more olive oil, fresh fruits and vegetables, whole grains, and fish into her diet while reducing red meat and processed foods. She also started enjoying a glass of red wine in moderation with her meals.

Results: Over the years, Maria's heart health improved significantly. Her cholesterol levels normalized, and she felt more energetic. Inspired by her success, Maria shared her journey with her family, and they collectively adopted a Mediterranean-inspired way of eating.

Case Study 2: Indigenous Diet Reclamation

Meet the Navajo Nation in the southwestern United States.

Background: The Navajo Nation faced high rates of diet-related health issues, including diabetes and obesity. Many residents sought to reconnect with their ancestral diet to address these concerns.

Application: Community leaders initiated efforts to revitalize traditional Navajo foods. This involved reintroducing foods like blue corn, squash, and wild game into daily meals. They also promoted traditional cooking techniques and shared knowledge among community members.

Results: Over time, the Navajo Nation witnessed improvements in health outcomes. Rates of diabetes and obesity began to decline, and community members reported feeling more connected to their cultural heritage through their dietary choices.

Case Study 3: The Return to African Heritage Foods

Meet Kwame, a Ghanaian immigrant living in the United Kingdom.

Background: Kwame had migrated to the UK but found himself missing the traditional foods of his homeland. He was also concerned about the impact of the Western diet on his health.

Application: Kwame sought out local markets and specialty stores to find ingredients that mirrored those from Ghana. He began cooking traditional dishes like jollof rice, fufu, and groundnut soup. He also incorporated more vegetables and whole grains into his meals.

Results: Kwame not only felt more connected to his cultural heritage but also experienced improvements in his overall health. His weight stabilized, and he had more energy. Kwame also formed a community of like-minded individuals who shared his passion for African cuisine.

Key Takeaways

These case studies underscore several important lessons:

- **Personalization:** Ancestral diets can be adapted to individual preferences and dietary needs, making them accessible and effective for various people.

- **Community Impact:** The successful adoption of ancestral diets often extends beyond individuals to positively impact families and communities.

- **Cultural Connection:** Embracing traditional foods fosters a deeper connection to one's cultural heritage and can be a source of pride and identity.

- **Health Benefits:** Ancestral diets can yield tangible health benefits, including improved heart health, reduced rates of chronic diseases, and enhanced overall well-being.

Case Study 4: Traditional Japanese Diet for Longevity

Meet Takeshi and Yuki, a retired couple living in Japan.

Background: Takeshi and Yuki had heard about the remarkable longevity of Japanese people and decided to embrace a traditional Japanese diet to improve their own health.

Application: They made several changes to their eating habits, following the principles of the traditional Japanese diet:

- **Fish and Seafood:** Takeshi and Yuki incorporated more fish and seafood into their meals, particularly fatty fish like salmon and mackerel.

- **Rice:** They switched from refined white rice to brown rice, which is richer in fiber and nutrients.

- **Vegetables:** Their plates were filled with a variety of seasonal vegetables, including leafy greens, seaweed, and daikon radish.

- **Fermented Foods:** They began consuming fermented foods like miso soup, natto (fermented soybeans), and pickles for gut health.

- **Tea:** Takeshi and Yuki replaced sugary beverages with green tea, a traditional Japanese staple known for its antioxidants.

Results: Over the years, Takeshi and Yuki experienced notable improvements in their health. They maintained a healthy weight, had lower cholesterol levels, and enjoyed a strong sense of vitality in their retirement years. Their commitment to the traditional Japanese diet not only enhanced their well-being but also inspired their children and grandchildren to adopt similar dietary habits.

Case Study 5: Paleo Diet for Autoimmune Health

Meet Sarah, a woman living in Australia.

Background: Sarah had been diagnosed with an autoimmune condition that caused chronic inflammation and fatigue. Determined to regain her health, she turned to the Paleo diet, which draws inspiration from the diets of our Paleolithic ancestors.

Application: Sarah eliminated processed foods, grains, dairy, and legumes from her diet, focusing instead on:

- **Lean Proteins:** She included ample servings of lean meats, poultry, and fish in her meals.

- **Vegetables:** Her plate was dominated by colorful vegetables, especially non-starchy varieties.

- **Healthy Fats:** Sarah embraced healthy fats like avocado, olive oil, and nuts.

- **Low Glycemic Fruits:** She enjoyed fruits in moderation, with an emphasis on those low in sugar.

- **Bone Broth:** Sarah incorporated bone broth into her diet to support gut health and reduce inflammation.

Results: Over time, Sarah's autoimmune symptoms significantly improved. She experienced less pain and inflammation and had more energy. While the Paleo diet required commitment and careful planning, it transformed Sarah's life by allowing her to manage her autoimmune condition effectively.

Key Takeaways

These additional case studies reinforce key takeaways:

- **Health Transformation:** Ancestral diets can lead to transformative improvements in health, particularly when addressing specific health conditions.

- **Sustainability:** Many individuals find that ancestral diets are sustainable and can become a long-term lifestyle choice.

- **Family Influence:** Individuals who experience health benefits often inspire their families and communities to embrace similar dietary practices.

- **Personalized Approaches:** Ancestral diets can be adapted to meet individual health goals and preferences, whether it's longevity, autoimmune health, or overall vitality.

Conclusion: The Power of Ancestral Wisdom

These case studies demonstrate the enduring power of ancestral wisdom in the realm of nutrition. They remind us that our dietary choices are not only about nourishing our bodies but also about preserving our heritage, fostering community, and achieving better health. By drawing inspiration from the diets of our ancestors, we can create a modern plate that reflects our roots while supporting our well-being.

54
MOVING FORWARD: NURTURING HEALTH WITH ANCESTRAL AND MODERN WISDOM

As we conclude our journey through the realms of ancestral and modern dietary wisdom, it's time to reflect on the lessons learned and chart a path forward that nurtures our health and well-being.

The Wisdom of Ancestral Diets

Throughout this book, we've explored the rich tapestry of ancestral diets from around the world. We've seen how these diets are steeped in tradition, shaped by local ecosystems, and intimately tied to cultural identities. Ancestral diets offer several enduring lessons:

- **Nutrient-Rich Whole Foods:** Across cultures, ancestral diets prioritize whole, unprocessed foods that provide a bounty of essential nutrients.

- **Seasonal and Local Eating:** Many ancestral diets revolve around the seasons, celebrating the availability of locally sourced ingredients.

- **Balanced Nutrition:** These diets naturally strike a balance of macronutrients and are rich in vitamins, minerals, and antioxidants.

- **Cultural Significance:** Food is more than sustenance; it's a reflection of cultural heritage and a source of community and identity.

The Realities of Modern Life

In our modern world, we face a different set of challenges:

- **Convenience Foods:** Processed and convenience foods have become ubiquitous, contributing to health concerns.

- **Fast-Paced Lifestyles:** Busy schedules often lead to less mindful eating and reliance on quick meals.

- **Globalization:** While it has expanded our culinary horizons, globalization can sometimes disconnect us from local and seasonal food sources.

Forging a Path Forward: Integrating Wisdom

To nurture our health with a blend of ancestral and modern wisdom, consider these steps:

- **Whole Foods:** Prioritize whole, unprocessed foods in your diet. These foods provide essential nutrients and minimize exposure to artificial additives.

- **Mindful Eating:** Cultivate mindful eating practices, savoring each bite and appreciating the sensory experience of food.

- **Local and Seasonal:** Whenever possible, choose local and seasonal produce. This supports local agriculture, reduces environmental impact, and provides fresher, more flavorful foods.

- **Cultural Heritage:** Explore your cultural heritage through food. Learn traditional recipes and cooking techniques that connect you with your roots.

- **Balanced Meals:** Strive for balanced meals that include a variety of foods and nutrients, reflecting the principles of ancestral diets.

A Holistic Approach

Remember that the pursuit of well-being is a holistic endeavor:

- **Physical Activity:** Regular exercise is essential for overall health.

- **Stress Management:** Stress can impact health; find techniques to manage it.

- **Supportive Relationships:** Connections with others contribute to emotional well-being.

Case Study: A Journey to Holistic Well-being

Meet Sarah, a working professional in her mid-30s.

Background: Sarah's life was characterized by the demands of a high-stress job, and she often found herself turning to processed foods and sugary snacks for comfort. She experienced fatigue, mood swings, and digestive issues, which significantly affected her overall well-being.

Turning Point: Sarah reached a turning point when she decided to take control of her health. Inspired by her grandmother's tales of traditional Indian cooking, she embarked on a journey to integrate ancestral wisdom into her modern lifestyle.

Application: Sarah made several changes to her daily routine:

- **Mindful Eating:** She began practicing mindful eating, taking the time to savor each bite and appreciate the flavors and textures of her meals.

- **Traditional Recipes:** Sarah started cooking traditional Indian dishes, incorporating a wide variety of spices, legumes, and vegetables into her meals.

- **Balanced Plate:** She aimed for a balanced plate, ensuring a mix of carbohydrates, proteins, and healthy fats.

- **Stress Management:** Sarah integrated stress-reduction techniques into her daily routine, including meditation and regular breaks during her workday.

Results: Over the course of several months, Sarah experienced remarkable improvements in her well-being. Her energy levels stabilized, digestive issues subsided, and her mood became more stable. She also found a sense of connection to her cultural heritage through her dietary choices.

Key Takeaways

Sarah's journey encapsulates the key takeaways from this book:

- **Personal Transformation:** Embracing ancestral wisdom can lead to profound personal transformations, improving both physical and emotional well-being.

- **Mindful Living:** Mindful eating and stress management are vital components of a holistic approach to health.

- **Cultural Connection:** Reconnecting with one's cultural heritage through food can be a source of pride and well-being.

Conclusion: Your Unique Journey

As you forge your path forward, remember that your journey to well-being is unique. It may draw inspiration from ancestral wisdom, cultural heritage, or individual dietary preferences. What matters most is the conscious effort to nourish your body and soul, fostering a harmonious and fulfilling life.

BONUS SECTION

The Symphony of Spices: Tracing Indian Food History and Culture

55

THE SYMPHONY OF SPICES: TRACING INDIAN FOOD HISTORY AND CULTURE

In our culinary exploration, we embark on a unique detour into the vibrant and diverse world of Indian cuisine, a tapestry of flavors, aromas, and traditions that have captivated palates for centuries. Indian food is not just about sustenance; it's a reflection of history, culture, geography, and the intricate interplay of spices and ingredients. Join us on this journey through the kaleidoscope of Indian food history and culture.

A Land of Culinary Diversity

India's culinary landscape is a testament to its incredible diversity. From the lush valleys of Kerala to the arid deserts of Rajasthan, every region boasts its own distinctive flavors and cooking techniques. The ingredients are as varied as the geography, with an array of grains, legumes, vegetables, and spices that form the foundation of Indian cuisine.

The Historical Tapestry

Indian food history is a tapestry woven through millennia. It traces its roots to the Indus Valley Civilization, where people cultivated wheat, barley, rice, and lentils. Over centuries, India saw the influence of Persian, Greek, and Central Asian cuisines through trade and conquests. The arrival of the Mughals in the 16th century brought an opulent and aromatic dimension to Indian cooking, with dishes like biryani and kebabs becoming iconic.

The Spice Route

Spices are the heartbeat of Indian cuisine, and the country's geographical location made it a hotspot for the spice trade. India has been a treasure trove of spices like cardamom, black pepper, cinnamon, and cloves, coveted by traders from around the world. The spice route not only enriched Indian cuisine but also played a pivotal role in shaping global culinary traditions.

A Symphony of Flavors

Indian cooking is a symphony of flavors, with each spice and ingredient contributing to the melody. The famous Indian spice blends, such as garam masala and curry powder, are a testament to the art of harmonizing diverse flavors. The balance of sweet, sour, salty, bitter, and umami is achieved through the skillful use of spices and seasonings.

Vegetarian Heritage

India's long-standing tradition of vegetarianism is deeply rooted in its cultural and religious history. Vegetarian dishes, such as dal (lentil stew), paneer (cottage cheese), and aloo gobi (potato and cauliflower curry), are staples in many Indian households. The concept of ahimsa, or non-violence, has also contributed to the prevalence of vegetarianism.

Regional Gems

Every region in India boasts its culinary gems. From the fiery vindaloo of Goa to the hearty saag paneer of Punjab, each state offers a unique culinary experience. The coastal regions are known for their seafood delicacies, while the north revels in rich gravies and tandoori delights.

Street Food Extravaganza

Indian street food is a sensory explosion. Chaat, samosas, dosas, and kebabs tempt passersby with their irresistible aromas and flavors. The bustling streets of cities like Mumbai and Delhi are veritable foodie paradises, where one can savor a world of tastes in a single stroll.

The Ritual of Meals

In Indian culture, a meal is not just a physical necessity; it's a ritual. The concept of "unity in diversity" is vividly expressed through communal dining, where people of various backgrounds come together to share a meal. Food in India is a bridge that connects people, fostering bonds and strengthening relationships.

A Cultural Kaleidoscope

Indian cuisine is not merely about taste; it's about storytelling. Each dish has a tale to tell, whether it's the royal history of biryani or the humble origins of street food. Indian food is also a reflection of festivals, rituals, and celebrations, with dishes tailored to specific occasions.

Preserving Tradition in a Modern World

In today's fast-paced world, Indian cuisine faces the challenge of preserving its traditions while embracing modernity. Contemporary Indian chefs are reimagining classic recipes with innovative twists, and Indian flavors are finding their way into global culinary trends.

Conclusion

The story of Indian food history and culture is a journey through time and taste, a voyage that encapsulates the essence of a nation's identity. It's a celebration of the culinary traditions that have stood the test of time, and a testament to the enduring power of spices, flavors, and the shared joy of a good meal. As we conclude this bonus chapter, let the symphony of spices and the richness of

Indian culture inspire your own culinary adventures. In every dish, you'll find a story waiting to be savored.

56
THE VEDIC PERIOD: A CULINARY BEGINNING

Our journey into the rich tapestry of Indian food history and culture begins with the Vedic period, a time of profound intellectual and spiritual awakening in ancient India. During this era, which spanned from approximately 1500 BCE to 500 BCE, the foundations of Indian cuisine, agricultural practices, and dietary norms were first laid down. Let's delve into the culinary wisdom of the Vedas and the significance of "Ahara" (diet) in the ancient Indian system of Ayurveda.

Ancient Texts and Culinary Insights

The Vedas, the oldest sacred scriptures of Hinduism, are a treasure trove of knowledge that offer valuable insights into the culinary practices of the time. These texts, composed in Sanskrit, provide a glimpse into the dietary choices, agricultural techniques, and food rituals of the Vedic period.

In the Rigveda, one of the oldest Vedic texts, we find references to the importance of grains, milk, and honey in the diet. Grains like barley and rice were staples, and milk was considered a symbol of purity and nourishment. Honey, known for its sweetness and medicinal properties, was also a prized ingredient.

The Significance of "Ahara" in Ayurveda

The concept of "Ahara" (diet) occupies a central place in Ayurveda, the ancient Indian system of medicine. Ayurveda, which means "the science of life," recognizes the profound connection between food and health. It emphasizes that the food we consume not only nourishes our bodies but also affects our overall well-being.

In Ayurveda, food is classified based on its taste (rasa), potency (virya), post-digestive effect (vipaka), and its impact on the three doshas—Vata, Pitta, and Kapha. The doshas are fundamental energies that govern our physical and mental constitution. The balance of these doshas is crucial for optimal health.

The Six Tastes (Shad Rasas)

Ayurveda recognizes six tastes, each with its unique qualities and effects on the body:

- **Sweet (Madhura):** This taste nourishes and soothes, promoting strength and vitality. It is found in foods like grains, fruits, and dairy products.

- **Sour (Amla):** Sour foods stimulate digestion and increase salivation. They include citrus fruits, yogurt, and fermented foods.

- **Salty (Lavana):** Salty foods improve taste perception and enhance digestion. Sea salt and certain vegetables fall into this category.

- **Bitter (Tikta):** Bitter foods detoxify and cool the body. They include leafy greens, bitter gourds, and turmeric.

- **Pungent (Katu):** Pungent foods promote circulation and stimulate digestion. Spices like chili peppers, garlic, and ginger belong to this category.

- **Astringent (Kashaya):** Astringent foods have a drying effect and can help balance excess moisture in the body. They include legumes, some fruits, and certain vegetables.

Balancing the Doshas

In Ayurveda, individuals are classified into different dosha types based on their physical and mental characteristics. By understanding their dosha constitution, people can tailor their diets to maintain balance and harmony within their bodies.

For example:

- Vata individuals, who tend to be energetic but easily overwhelmed, benefit from warm, nourishing foods and gentle spices to calm their restless nature.

- Pitta individuals, who are fiery and competitive, thrive on cooling, hydrating foods and mild spices to pacify their inner fire.

- Kapha individuals, who are steady but prone to sluggishness, benefit from light, spicy foods and warming spices to invigorate their energy.

Conclusion

The Vedic period and the wisdom of Ayurveda laid the groundwork for the intricate and holistic approach to food and health that continues to influence Indian cuisine and dietary practices to this day. The concept of "Ahara" as a vital component of Ayurveda underscores the profound connection between what we eat and how we feel. As we journey through the chapters of Indian food history and culture, we'll uncover the evolution of these culinary principles and their enduring impact on the diverse and flavorful world of Indian cuisine.

57
THE MUGHAL IMPACT

In the annals of Indian culinary history, few chapters are as influential and transformative as the advent of the Mughals. With their arrival in the Indian subcontinent in the early 16th century, the Mughals brought with them a rich tapestry of flavors, ingredients, and culinary techniques that forever altered the course of Indian cuisine. Let's delve into how the Mughals reshaped Indian gastronomy, introducing new ingredients, techniques, and dishes, and explore the fascinating amalgamation of Indian and Persian culinary practices.

A Culinary Renaissance

The Mughals, descendants of Genghis Khan and Timur, were renowned for their opulent lifestyles and appreciation for the finer things in life. This included a deep passion for exquisite food and the culinary arts. When Babur, the founder of the Mughal Empire in India, set foot on the subcontinent in 1526, he brought Persian chefs and culinary traditions that would leave an indelible mark on Indian cuisine.

Influences and Ingredients

Persian and Central Asian Influences: Mughal cuisine bore the indelible imprint of Persian and Central Asian culinary traditions. Techniques such as slow-cooking in tandoors (clay ovens) and the use of aromatic spices and dried fruits found their way into Mughal kitchens.

Exotic Ingredients: The Mughals introduced a wealth of new ingredients to the Indian palate, including saffron, dried fruits like raisins and apricots, and Persian herbs like mint and coriander. These ingredients added depth and complexity to Indian dishes.

The Mughal Kitchen

The Mughal kitchen was a theater of culinary excellence. Royal chefs, known as "bawarchis," crafted intricate dishes that blended the flavors of India and Persia. The "Nauratan Korma," a dish made with nine types of meats, exemplifies the opulence of Mughal feasting.

Biryani and Kebabs

Two enduring legacies of Mughal cuisine are biryani and kebabs. Biryani, a fragrant rice dish, was developed from the Persian "pilaf" and combined with Indian spices and flavors. Kebabs, such as seekh kebabs and shami kebabs, became synonymous with Mughal dining, showcasing the art of marination and skewer-grilling.

Influence on Vegetarian Cuisine

Even though the Mughals were known for their love of meat, their culinary influence extended to vegetarian dishes as well. Dishes like "navratan korma" (a creamy vegetable stew) and "paneer tikka" (grilled cottage cheese) exemplify their innovative approach to vegetarian cooking.

The Royal Legacy

The Mughal emperors were connoisseurs of fine dining, and their patronage of culinary arts elevated Indian cuisine to new heights. They hosted extravagant feasts, "darbars," where gastronomic

delights were celebrated with music and poetry. The famous
"Akbari Khana," a royal recipe book, documented the culinary
legacy of Emperor Akbar.

The Synthesis of Cultures

The Mughal influence was not merely about Persian ingredients
and techniques; it was a fusion of cultures. It blended Persian
refinement with Indian exuberance, resulting in a culinary
landscape that celebrated diversity and innovation. This synthesis
of cultures laid the foundation for the rich and varied Indian
cuisine we know today.

Conclusion

The Mughal era was a golden age of culinary creativity in India,
where the confluence of Indian and Persian influences birthed a
gastronomic renaissance. The introduction of new ingredients,
techniques, and dishes transformed Indian cuisine, enriching it with
the opulence and sophistication that continue to define it to this
day. As we journey through the chapters of Indian food history
and culture, we'll uncover how subsequent generations built upon
the Mughal legacy, creating a culinary heritage that is as diverse as it
is delectable.

58

SPICE TRADE AND GLOBAL INFLUENCES

India's influence on world cuisine extends far beyond its borders, and at the heart of this culinary exchange lies the spice trade. For centuries, India was a spice powerhouse, exporting fragrant and exotic spices to the far reaches of the globe. This trade not only shaped Indian cuisine but also left an indelible mark on world cooking. In this chapter, we delve into India's pivotal role in the global spice trade and how it influenced world cuisine. We also explore how external influences were seamlessly integrated into Indian cooking, creating a culinary mosaic that continues to dazzle palates worldwide.

The Spice Trade: India's Fragrant Legacy

India's association with spices dates back over 7,000 years, with references to spices found in ancient texts like the Rigveda. The spice trade was a source of wealth and power for Indian empires, attracting traders from as far as Rome and China.

Spices as Currency: Spices were so highly prized that they often served as currency in trade. Pepper, known as "black gold," was a particularly valuable commodity, with trade routes collectively called the "Pepper Route" or "Spice Route."

The Spread of Indian Spices: Indian spices like black pepper, cardamom, cinnamon, cloves, and ginger traveled across Asia, the Middle East, and Europe, where they became essential ingredients in regional cuisines.

The Impact on World Cuisine

Arab and Persian Influences: India's proximity to the Middle East facilitated the exchange of culinary ideas. Persian influences, such as the use of dried fruits, nuts, and saffron, found their way into Mughal and Indian cooking.

The Birth of Fusion Cuisine: The arrival of European powers, including the Portuguese, Dutch, and British, in India led to the fusion of Indian and European cuisines. Dishes like "Vindaloo" and "Curry" are examples of this cross-cultural exchange.

The Spice That Launched Explorations: The quest for Indian spices, particularly pepper and cloves, was one of the driving forces behind European exploration, leading to the discovery of new lands and the Columbian Exchange.

Integration of Global Ingredients

Indian-Chinese Fusion: The Chinese influence on Indian cuisine is evident in dishes like "Manchurian" and "Chow Mein," which blend Indian spices with Chinese cooking techniques.

Influence of Southeast Asia: India's trade links with Southeast Asia resulted in the adoption of ingredients like coconut, tamarind, and galangal in Indian coastal cuisines.

The Global Curry: The term "curry" is derived from the Tamil word "kari," which means sauce. It became a convenient way for Europeans to describe the diverse and complex dishes they encountered in India.

Spices in World History

The Spice Wars: The competition for control over spice-producing regions led to conflicts and the rise of colonial empires.

European powers sought to dominate the spice trade for its economic and strategic value.

The Columbian Exchange: The exchange of crops and spices between the Old World (Asia, Africa, and Europe) and the New World (the Americas) during the Age of Exploration transformed global cuisines. Spices like chili peppers, vanilla, and cacao enriched culinary traditions on both sides of the Atlantic.

Conclusion

The story of India's role in the global spice trade is a testament to the enduring allure of spices and their capacity to transcend borders and cultures. India's culinary gifts to the world have enriched countless cuisines and continue to be celebrated for their flavor and fragrance. As we explore the chapters of Indian food history and culture, we'll unravel more tales of culinary exchange and the magic of spices that connect us all.

59
SPIRITUALITY AND CULINARY PRACTICES

India's spiritual and culinary landscapes are intertwined in a profound and intricate dance. The country's diverse spiritual beliefs, including Hinduism, Buddhism, and Jainism, have deeply influenced food habits, elevating the act of eating into a sacred ritual. In this chapter, we'll unpack the interplay between India's spiritual beliefs and food practices, examining the philosophy behind vegetarianism and the sacredness of food.

Hinduism: The Vegetarian Way

Hinduism, one of the world's oldest religions, has a significant impact on Indian culinary traditions. Central to Hindu dietary practices is the principle of "ahimsa," or non-violence. Many Hindus embrace vegetarianism as a means to live in harmony with the universe and avoid causing harm to other living beings.

Sacred Cows: The cow holds a special place in Hinduism and is revered as a symbol of divine and natural beneficence. This sacred status has led to the widespread practice of vegetarianism among Hindus.

Vegetarian Feast: Hindu cuisine is a treasure trove of vegetarian delights, with a myriad of dishes made from grains, legumes, vegetables, and dairy products. Dishes like "paneer tikka," "dal makhani," and "aloo gobi" are beloved by vegetarians and non-vegetarians alike.

Buddhism: Mindful Eating

Buddhism, born in India, advocates mindful and compassionate living, which extends to dietary choices. While not all Buddhists are vegetarians, many follow a vegetarian or vegan diet to practice non-harming and mindfulness.

Monastic Meals: Buddhist monks and nuns adhere to strict dietary rules, including eating only what is offered to them and avoiding foods that involve the killing of animals.

Jainism: The Ultimate Non-Violence

Jainism takes the principle of non-violence to its highest level. Jains believe in the sanctity of all life forms, and their dietary choices reflect this belief. The Jain diet is one of the most restrictive vegetarian diets in the world.

Ahimsa and Anekantavada: Ahimsa (non-violence) is central to Jainism, and followers avoid eating root vegetables and foods with a high likelihood of containing microorganisms. The philosophy of "anekantavada" emphasizes the multiplicity of viewpoints, which also informs their approach to food.

The Sacredness of Food

In India, food is not merely sustenance; it is an offering, a connection to the divine, and a means to elevate one's consciousness.

Prasad: In Hindu temples, food offered to deities is distributed as "prasad" to devotees. Consuming prasad is believed to impart blessings and spiritual nourishment.

Fasting: Fasting is a common spiritual practice in India. Whether it's during religious festivals or specific days of the week, fasting is seen as a way to purify the body and mind.

Sattvic Diet: In Ayurveda, there is a concept of "sattvic" food, which is pure, nourishing, and conducive to spiritual growth. It includes fruits, vegetables, grains, and dairy products.

Conclusion

In India, spirituality and food are intertwined, creating a tapestry of culinary practices that reflect profound beliefs about non-violence, mindfulness, and the sacredness of life. The diverse spiritual traditions of Hinduism, Buddhism, and Jainism have left an indelible mark on Indian cuisine, fostering a reverence for nature, life, and the act of eating itself. As we journey through the chapters of Indian food history and culture, we'll continue to explore how these beliefs have shaped India's culinary tapestry and influenced the dietary choices of its people.

60
REGIONAL DIVERSITIES

India is a vast and diverse land, and its culinary landscape is a reflection of this rich tapestry of cultures, climates, and landscapes. Each region of India boasts its own unique flavors, ingredients, and cooking techniques, resulting in a culinary mosaic that is as diverse as it is delectable. In this chapter, we embark on a culinary journey across the length and breadth of India, exploring the regional cuisines, signature dishes, cooking techniques, and staple ingredients that make each state's culinary tradition a feast for the senses.

North India: Aromatic Indulgence

- **Punjab:** Known as the "Land of Five Rivers," Punjab's cuisine is a celebration of hearty flavors. Signature dishes include "butter chicken," "sarson da saag" (mustard greens), and "makki di roti" (cornflat bread).

- **Kashmir:** In the scenic valleys of Kashmir, you'll find the fragrant "rogan josh," "gushtaba," and the beloved "yakhni" - dishes that showcase the region's love for aromatic spices and yogurt-based gravies.

West India: Spice and Seafood

- **Gujarat:** Gujarat's cuisine is a delightful blend of sweet, spicy, and tangy flavors. "Dhokla," "khandvi," and "thepla" are popular snacks, while "undhiyu" is a beloved winter dish.

- **Maharashtra:** Maharashtra's coastal location infuses its cuisine with an abundance of seafood. "Vada pav," "misal pav," and "puran poli" are cherished dishes, showcasing a balance of spices and textures.

East India: Fresh and Flavorful

- **Bengal:** Bengal's cuisine is famous for its love of fish. "Machher jhol" (fish curry), "shorshe ilish" (hilsa fish in mustard sauce), and "rasgulla" are iconic dishes that exemplify the region's culinary finesse.

- **Odisha:** Odisha's cuisine emphasizes simple yet flavorful vegetarian dishes like "dalma," "bhendi bhaja" (fried okra), and "pakhala" (fermented rice). Seafood lovers also relish "chhena poda," a cheese dessert.

South India: A Symphony of Spices

- **Tamil Nadu:** Tamil Nadu's cuisine is known for its fiery and flavorful dishes like "chettinad chicken curry," "idli," "dosai," and "sambar."

- **Kerala:** Kerala's cuisine features an abundance of coconut and seafood. "Appam," "avial," and "karimeen pollichathu" (spiced fish) are must-try dishes.

Central India: Hearty and Spicy

- **Madhya Pradesh:** Madhya Pradesh's cuisine is characterized by its use of wheat, maize, and jowar. "Poha," "bafla," and "bhutte ka kees" (corn-based dish) are popular.

- **Chhattisgarh:** Chhattisgarh's cuisine highlights the use of rice and a variety of lentils. "Chana samosa," "chana jhor," and "bore baasi" (sun-dried lentil dumplings) are notable dishes.

Northeast India: Exotic and Eclectic

- **Assam:** Assam's cuisine features bold and aromatic flavors. "Assam laksa," "bamboo shoot curry," and "masor tenga" (sour fish curry) are culinary delights.

- **Nagaland:** Nagaland's cuisine is known for its use of smoked and fermented ingredients. "Smoked pork curry," "bamboo shoot chutney," and "axone" (fermented soybean) are unique to the region.

Conclusion

India's regional cuisines are a testament to the country's culinary diversity, with each state offering a distinct and flavorful experience. From the fiery spices of the South to the hearty flavors of the North, and the exotic ingredients of the Northeast, India's regional cuisines reflect the depth and complexity of its cultural tapestry. As we explore the chapters of Indian food history and culture, we'll continue to savor the richness of these regional traditions, discovering the essence of India's culinary identity in every bite.

61

COLONIAL INFLUENCES

India's culinary heritage is a melting pot of diverse flavors, and its history of colonization by the British and Portuguese has significantly contributed to this tapestry. The colonial era brought with it not only new crops and ingredients but also a culinary exchange that birthed unique dishes. In this chapter, we delve into the culinary impacts of British and Portuguese colonization, exploring the introduction of new crops and the fusion of Indian and colonial influences in dishes like Railway Mutton Curry and Vindaloo.

British Colonialism: A Culinary Exchange

The British colonization of India, which lasted for over two centuries, had a profound impact on the country's culinary landscape.

Introduction of New Crops: The British introduced crops like tea, coffee, potatoes, and various fruits to India, some of which are now staples in Indian cuisine.

Anglo-Indian Cuisine: The fusion of British and Indian culinary traditions gave rise to Anglo-Indian cuisine. Dishes like "mulligatawny soup," "cutlets," and "bread and butter pudding" are examples of this blend.

Railway Mutton Curry: This iconic dish has its origins in the British colonial period. It was created to cater to British officers traveling on India's extensive railway network. Today, it remains a beloved part of Indian cuisine, known for its rich and spicy tomato-based gravy.

Portuguese Colonial Influence: The Vindaloo Legacy

Portuguese explorers arrived in India in the 16th century, bringing with them a love for spices and a culinary tradition that would leave a lasting mark.

Vindaloo: The famous dish "vindaloo" has its roots in Portuguese cuisine. Originally "carne de vinha d'alhos," it was a dish of marinated meat cooked with wine and garlic. In India, it underwent transformation with the addition of local spices, especially red chilies and vinegar. Today, vindaloo is known for its fiery and tangy flavor.

Chili Peppers: The introduction of chili peppers by the Portuguese revolutionized Indian cuisine. These fiery peppers quickly became an integral part of many Indian dishes.

The Culinary Tapestry of Goa: Goa, a former Portuguese colony, boasts a unique blend of Indian and Portuguese flavors. Dishes like "sorpotel," "bebinca," and "balchão" are emblematic of this fusion.

Cultural Exchange Through Food

The colonial era was not just about the exchange of ingredients; it was also a time of cultural exchange.

High Tea: The British tradition of "high tea" made its way to India, leading to the popularity of tea as an essential part of Indian culture.

Cultural Fusion: The blending of culinary traditions also led to the emergence of new dishes and flavors that continue to captivate taste buds around the world.

Conclusion

The colonial influences on Indian cuisine have left an indelible mark, enriching it with new ingredients, techniques, and flavors. The British introduced crops that have become staples, and the Portuguese left behind a fiery and flavorful legacy, best embodied by vindaloo. The culinary exchanges that occurred during this period have not only shaped India's cuisine but also added to the cultural richness of the nation. As we explore the chapters of Indian food history and culture, we'll continue to uncover the layers of influence that have made Indian cuisine a global sensation.

$$62$$

FESTIVALS AND FOOD

India is a land of festivals, and each festival comes with its own unique culinary delights. From sweets that symbolize prosperity to savory dishes that commemorate historical events, Indian festivals are a celebration of culture, tradition, and, of course, food. In this chapter, we dive into the numerous Indian festivals and the diverse array of foods associated with each celebration. We'll also explore the symbolism and cultural narratives that make festive foods an integral part of the festivities.

Diwali: The Festival of Lights

Diwali, also known as Deepavali, is one of India's most celebrated festivals, and it's synonymous with an abundance of sweets and snacks.

Sweets: "Gulab jamun," "jalebi," "ladoo," and "kaju katli" are just a few of the delectable sweets prepared during Diwali. These sweet treats symbolize the sweetness of life and the victory of light over darkness.

Savories: "Chivda," "mathri," and "namak para" are savory snacks enjoyed during Diwali, often exchanged among friends and family.

Holi: The Festival of Colors

Holi is a vibrant celebration marked by the throwing of colorful powders, and it's also a time for indulging in a range of special dishes.

Gujiya: These sweet dumplings, filled with khoya (milk solids), dry fruits, and cardamom, are a Holi staple. They symbolize the spirit of festivity and joy.

Bhang: In some regions, a special drink called "bhang" is prepared from cannabis leaves and consumed during Holi for its mood-enhancing properties.

Eid: The Festival of Feasts

Eid al-Fitr and Eid al-Adha are two major Muslim festivals celebrated with grand feasts.

Biryani: Eid is synonymous with the aroma of biryani wafting through households. The fragrant rice dish is often prepared with succulent pieces of meat.

Sheer Khurma: A rich and creamy dessert made with vermicelli, milk, and dates, sheer khurma is a symbol of festivity and is often served as a sweet ending to the feast.

Pongal: The Harvest Festival

Pongal, celebrated predominantly in South India, is a harvest festival dedicated to the Sun God.

Pongal Dish: The festival takes its name from a special dish called "Pongal," made from freshly harvested rice, lentils, and spices, cooked together in a clay pot. It symbolizes gratitude for the harvest and abundance.

Makar Sankranti: The Kite Festival

Makar Sankranti marks the transition of the sun into the zodiac sign of Capricorn and is celebrated with the exchange of sesame and jaggery sweets.

Tilgul: "Tilgul" are sweet sesame seed and jaggery laddoos exchanged with the phrase "Tilgul ghya, god god bola" ("Accept these tilguls and speak sweet words").

Symbolism and Unity

Festive foods in India are more than just delicious; they carry deep cultural and symbolic significance.

Unity and Togetherness: Festive meals often bring families and communities together, reinforcing bonds and sharing the joy of the occasion.

Symbolism of Ingredients: The choice of ingredients in festive foods often reflects cultural narratives and historical events, making the act of eating a way to connect with the past.

Conclusion

Indian festivals are a kaleidoscope of colors, traditions, and flavors. The diverse array of foods associated with each celebration adds a unique dimension to the festivities, conveying messages of prosperity, togetherness, and cultural continuity. As we explore the chapters of Indian food history and culture, we'll continue to savor the richness of these culinary traditions and the stories they tell about India's vibrant cultural tapestry.

63

INDIAN STREET FOOD CULTURE

India's bustling streets are a gastronomic paradise, offering a vast array of flavors and culinary experiences. Street food is an integral part of Indian culture, a delightful fusion of taste, tradition, and convenience. In this chapter, we embark on a journey to investigate the vibrant street food culture across different regions of India. We'll explore popular snacks, beverages, and quick meals, understanding their roots and sociocultural importance.

North India: Chaat and Beyond

- **Chaat:** This iconic North Indian street food is a medley of crispy fried dough, tangy tamarind chutney, spicy seasonings, and cool yogurt. Varieties like "aloo tikki chaat," "papdi chaat," and "raj kachori" are beloved snacks.

- **Kulfi:** A traditional Indian ice cream, kulfi comes in various flavors like pistachio, rose, and saffron, served on sticks or in earthen pots.

South India: Dosa and More

- **Dosa:** A thin, crispy rice crepe, dosa is often served with coconut chutney and spicy sambar. Variations like "masala dosa" (filled with potato masala) are immensely popular.

- **Idli:** Soft, steamed rice cakes, idlis are a nutritious breakfast option, often paired with coconut chutney and tomato-based sambar.

West India: Vada Pav and Beyond

- **Vada Pav:** Often referred to as the Indian burger, vada pav consists of a spicy potato fritter enclosed in a bun. It's a quintessential street snack in Mumbai.

- **Pav Bhaji:** This spicy vegetable curry served with buttery rolls is a hearty and filling street food dish.

East India: Momos and Beyond

- **Momos:** Originally from Tibet, momos have found a special place in the hearts of Indians. These steamed or fried dumplings are typically served with a spicy dipping sauce.

- **Puchka/Pani Puri:** Known by different names in different regions, these hollow, crispy spheres filled with spicy tamarind water, potato, and chickpeas are a must-try.

Rajasthan: Mirchi Bada and More

- **Mirchi Bada:** This spicy street snack features green chilies stuffed with spicy potato filling, dipped in gram flour batter, and deep-fried.

- **Kachori:** A deep-fried, flaky pastry filled with lentils or spices, kachori is often enjoyed with tamarind chutney.

Conclusion

Indian street food culture is a vibrant tapestry of flavors, reflecting the diversity of the nation's regions and culinary traditions. These quick and affordable meals not only satisfy the taste buds but also play a significant role in the sociocultural fabric of India. Street food vendors are often the storytellers of a city's history and heritage, and the street corners become stages where culinary traditions are passed down through generations. As we explore the chapters of Indian food history and culture, we'll continue to savor the richness of these street food experiences and the stories they tell about India's culinary landscape.

64

MODERN INDIAN CUISINE

Indian cuisine has evolved over centuries, and in recent years, it has undergone a transformation that transcends borders. Modern Indian cuisine isn't confined to traditional recipes but embraces innovation, fusion, and global influences. In this chapter, we examine contemporary trends in Indian cooking, both domestically and internationally. We'll discuss the global proliferation of Indian cuisine and its modern adaptations.

Domestic Evolution: Fusion and Innovation

Fusion Cuisine: Contemporary Indian chefs are known for their creativity in blending Indian flavors with international ingredients and cooking techniques. Dishes like "butter chicken pizza," "sushi with Indian spices," and "tandoori tacos" showcase this fusion trend.

Elevated Dining: Modern Indian restaurants are pushing culinary boundaries, offering fine dining experiences that showcase Indian flavors in innovative ways. These establishments are not only about food but also about artistry and presentation.

Health and Wellness: There's a growing focus on healthier cooking methods and ingredients in India, with traditional spices and herbs being recognized for their medicinal properties.

Global Proliferation: Indian Cuisine Worldwide

Indian Restaurants Abroad: Indian restaurants have found a global audience, from family-run eateries to Michelin-starred establishments. Cities like London, New York, and Dubai are hubs for Indian culinary experiences.

International Influences: Indian cuisine has influenced global culinary trends, with spices like turmeric and flavors like curry becoming pantry staples worldwide.

Modern Adaptations: International chefs are embracing Indian flavors and techniques, incorporating them into their own cuisines. This cross-pollination has led to unique culinary creations.

Conclusion

Modern Indian cuisine is a testament to the adaptability and timelessness of Indian flavors. It has evolved beyond its traditional boundaries, offering a dynamic and exciting culinary journey. Whether you're savoring innovative dishes in India or experiencing the global spread of Indian cuisine, you're sure to encounter the rich tapestry of flavors that make it a beloved and enduring culinary tradition. As we explore the chapters of Indian food history and culture, we'll continue to unravel the vibrant threads of contemporary Indian cuisine and its impact on the culinary world.

65 SUSTAINABLE AND HEALTHFUL PRACTICES

Traditional Indian diets are not just about flavor; they also embody principles of sustainability and healthfulness that have sustained generations. In this chapter, we'll delve into the inherent sustainability and healthful qualities of traditional Indian diets, as well as explore how Ayurvedic principles in diet promote overall wellbeing.

Sustainable Eating Practices

Seasonal Eating: Traditional Indian diets prioritize seasonal and locally sourced ingredients. This not only ensures freshness but also reduces the carbon footprint associated with long-distance transportation.

Plant-Based Focus: Indian cuisine features an abundance of vegetarian and vegan dishes. The emphasis on plant-based diets contributes to lower environmental impacts and reduced strain on natural resources.

Zero Waste Cooking: Many Indian dishes are designed to minimize food waste by using all parts of ingredients, such as stems, leaves, and peels.

Healthful Eating Practices

Ayurvedic Principles: Ayurveda, the ancient Indian system of medicine, places a strong emphasis on diet as a means of achieving and maintaining balance in the body. Ayurvedic principles promote a personalized approach to nutrition based on one's constitution (dosha) and the seasons.

Spices and Herbs: Indian cuisine incorporates a wide variety of spices and herbs, many of which have recognized health benefits. Turmeric, for example, is known for its anti-inflammatory properties, while spices like cumin aid digestion.

Balanced Meals: Traditional Indian meals are often a balance of carbohydrates, proteins, and fiber. Dishes like "dal" (lentils), "roti" (flatbread), and a variety of vegetables provide a well-rounded nutrient profile.

Mindful Eating: Indian culture encourages mindful eating practices, such as eating slowly, savoring flavors, and being present during meals. This can lead to better digestion and a healthier relationship with food.

Community and Connection: Shared meals and communal dining are integral to Indian culture. These practices promote not only physical nourishment but also emotional and social wellbeing.

Conclusion

Traditional Indian diets are a testament to the harmonious relationship between food, sustainability, and health. The incorporation of Ayurvedic principles and a focus on balanced, plant-based meals make Indian cuisine a holistic approach to nourishment. As we explore the chapters of Indian food history and culture, we'll continue to uncover the wisdom embedded in these dietary practices and their profound impact on personal and planetary wellbeing.

CONCLUSION

CONCLUSION I:
A CULINARY ODYSSEY - BRIDGING PAST AND PRESENT NAME

In the final pages of our culinary odyssey, we stand at the crossroads of the past and the present, carrying with us the knowledge and wisdom we've gathered on this enriching journey through the world of food, culture, and well-being. As we close this book, let's take a moment to reflect on the profound lessons we've unearthed and the path that lies ahead.

The Tapestry of Ancestral Wisdom

We began our journey by delving into the tapestry of ancestral diets, where we discovered that food is more than mere sustenance; it's a reflection of culture, history, and the ingenious adaptations of communities to their environments. We learned that the wisdom of our ancestors, passed down through generations, continues to hold invaluable insights into nourishing our bodies and souls.

Global Plates: A Journey Through Culinary Cultures

Our voyage took us on a global expedition, exploring the rich and diverse culinary traditions of cultures near and far. From the bustling street food stalls of Bangkok to the tranquil tea ceremonies of Japan, we marveled at the ways in which food serves as a bridge to connect people, customs, and the essence of a place. Through each culinary culture, we unearthed the universality of shared meals, the power of spices and flavors, and the beauty of preserving tradition in a rapidly changing world.

The Modern Plate: Food, Fitness, and Well-being

We confronted the challenges of modern life head-on, acknowledging the convenience-driven culture that often distances us from the wisdom of our ancestors. Yet, we also discovered that the integration of ancestral and modern wisdom is not only possible but profoundly transformative. We celebrated individuals and communities who revitalized their health, reconnected with their roots, and fostered well-being by embracing the principles of ancestral diets in their modern lives.

Your Journey to Wholeness

As we conclude our journey, we leave you with a sense of empowerment and possibility. Your own odyssey is just beginning, and your path to wholeness is uniquely yours to shape. Here are some parting thoughts to carry with you:

- **Nourishment Beyond the Plate:** Remember that nourishment extends beyond the plate. It includes the joy of sharing meals with loved ones, the tranquility of a mindful moment with a cup of tea, and the vitality that arises from a balanced life.

- **Cultural Connection:** Embrace your cultural heritage through food. The recipes and traditions passed down through generations can be a source of pride and a bridge to your roots.

- **Mindful Living:** Incorporate mindfulness into your daily life, from the way you eat to the way you manage stress.

These practices enhance not only your physical health but
also your emotional well-being.

- **Holistic Well-being:** Recognize that well-being is a
  holistic concept. It encompasses physical health, mental
  clarity, emotional resilience, and the nourishment of your
  spirit.

Your Future Plate

As you move forward, your future plate is a canvas waiting to be
painted with vibrant flavors, meaningful connections, and a deep
sense of well-being. It's a plate that reflects the wisdom of the past,
the practicality of the present, and the promise of the future.

In the end, our culinary odyssey is not just a journey through food;
it's a journey through life itself. It's a testament to the enduring
power of tradition, the limitless possibilities of modernity, and the
timeless quest for a life well-lived.

As you embark on your own culinary odyssey, may your future
plates be filled with nourishment, joy, and a deep sense of
connection to the world and the generations that have come
before. Bon appétit, and may your journey be as fulfilling as the
feast that life has to offer.

CONCLUSION II
THE ROLE OF TECHNOLOGY IN FOOD AND FITNESS

As we wrap up our exploration of the dynamic world of food and fitness, it's imperative to acknowledge the significant role that technology plays in shaping our modern lives, from the way we nourish our bodies to how we stay active and monitor our well-being. In this concluding chapter, we'll delve into the intersection of technology with food and fitness, highlighting both the promises and the challenges it presents.

The Technological Revolution

We are living in an era of unprecedented technological innovation. Our smartphones, wearable fitness trackers, and smart kitchen appliances have become integral parts of our daily routines. These technological advances have the potential to revolutionize the way we approach food and fitness, offering us new tools and insights to enhance our well-being.

Food and Technology

- **Access to Information:** Technology has granted us instant access to a wealth of information about nutrition, recipes, and dietary recommendations. Apps and websites provide nutritional data, meal planning tools, and recipe inspiration at our fingertips.

- **Food Delivery:** On-demand food delivery services and meal kit subscriptions have transformed the way we access and prepare meals. They offer convenience and variety, but also raise questions about the sustainability of food delivery systems.

- **Precision Nutrition:** Personalized nutrition is on the horizon, with advancements in genetic testing and data analysis. Soon, we may see diets tailored to individual genetic profiles and health goals.

- **Food Safety:** Technology aids in food safety through traceability systems, ensuring that the food we consume is of high quality and free from contaminants.

Fitness and Technology

- **Wearable Devices:** Fitness trackers and smartwatches provide real-time data on physical activity, heart rate, and sleep patterns. They encourage us to be more mindful of our activity levels and health metrics.

- **Virtual Workouts:** Online platforms and apps offer a wide range of virtual workouts, enabling us to exercise from the comfort of our homes. They also facilitate access to expert trainers and fitness communities.

- **Health Monitoring:** Technology allows for remote health monitoring, making it easier for individuals with chronic conditions to manage their health. Telehealth services have surged, providing greater accessibility to healthcare professionals.

- **Data Analytics:** The collection and analysis of health data empower individuals to make informed decisions about their fitness and well-being. However, data privacy and security concerns persist.

The Promise and the Balance

While technology has brought remarkable advances to our plates and our workouts, it's essential to strike a balance. Here are some key considerations:

- **Human Connection:** Technology should complement, not replace, the human connection in food and fitness. Shared meals, group exercise, and supportive communities remain essential.

- **Data Privacy:** As we embrace technology, safeguarding our personal health data is paramount. Robust privacy measures are crucial to protect our sensitive information.

- **Sustainability:** The environmental impact of technology, especially in the food industry, is a growing concern. We must seek sustainable solutions that minimize waste and energy consumption.

- **Moderation:** The convenience of technology should not lead to sedentary lifestyles or overreliance on processed foods. Balance is key to maintaining our health and vitality.

The Future of Food, Fitness, and Technology

The future holds boundless possibilities at the intersection of food, fitness, and technology. From AI-powered dietary recommendations to virtual reality fitness experiences, the landscape is ever-evolving.

As we navigate this technologically infused era, let's remain mindful of our choices and their impact on our well-being. Let's harness the power of technology to enhance our lives while preserving the essential elements of human connection, cultural heritage, and sustainability. Together, we can embrace the best of both worlds, where ancestral wisdom meets modern innovation, creating a brighter, healthier future.

In closing, let's embark on this journey with curiosity, discernment, and a deep appreciation for the intricate tapestry of food, fitness, and technology that shapes our lives. The future is bright, and the path to well-being is ever-evolving. May your pursuit of health and vitality be guided by wisdom, balance, and the enduring spirit of discovery.

REFERENCES

- *"The Paleo Diet" by Loren Cordain*
- *"The Primal Blueprint" by Mark Sisson*
- *"The Omnivore's Dilemma" by Michael Pollan*
- *"Nourishing Traditions" by Sally Fallon*
- *"Good Calories, Bad Calories" by Gary Taubes*
- *"In Defense of Food" by Michael Pollan*
- *"Sapiens: A Brief History of Humankind" by Yuval Noah Harari*
- *"The Blue Zones" by Dan Buettner*
- *"The China Study" by T. Colin Campbell*
- *"The 4-Hour Body" by Timothy Ferriss*
- *"Born to Run" by Christopher McDougall*
- *"Deep Nutrition" by Catherine Shanahan*
- *"The Bulletproof Diet" by Dave Asprey*
- *"The Art and Science of Low Carbohydrate Living" by Stephen D. Phinney and Jeff S. Volek*
- *"The Big Fat Surprise" by Nina Teicholz*

- *"Wired to Eat"* by Robb Wolf
- *"The Story of the Human Body"* by Daniel Lieberman
- *"The End of Food"* by Thomas F. Pawlick
- *"Salt Sugar Fat"* by Michael Moss
- *"Grain Brain"* by David Perlmutter
- *"The Jungle Effect"* by Daphne Miller
- *"The Botany of Desire"* by Michael Pollan
- *"Cooked: A Natural History of Transformation"* by Michael Pollan
- *"The Dorito Effect"* by Mark Schatzker
- *"The Lean Startup"* by Eric Ries (for insights on applying principles to health)
- *"The Wahls Protocol"* by Terry Wahls, M.D.
- *"The Plant Paradox"* by Steven R. Gundry, M.D.
- *"The Mind-Gut Connection"* by Emeran Mayer, M.D.
- *"Why We Get Fat"* by Gary Taubes
- *"The Genius of Flexibility"* by Bob Cooley
- *"The Hormone Reset Diet"* by Sara Gottfried, M.D.
- *"The Wild Diet"* by Abel James
- *"The Bulletproof Diet"* by Dave Asprey
- *"Healthy at 100"* by John Robbins
- *"Ancient Bodies, Modern Lives"* by Wenda Trevathan
- *"The Whole30"* by Melissa Hartwig and Dallas Hartwig
- *"The Longevity Diet"* by Valter Longo
- *"The Obesity Code"* by Dr. Jason Fung
- *"The Keto Reset Diet"* by Mark Sisson
- *"Super Genes"* by Deepak Chopra and Rudolph E. Tanzi
- *"The Plant-Based Solution"* by Joel K. Kahn, M.D.

- *"Gut: The Inside Story of Our Body's Most Underrated Organ" by Giulia Enders*
- *"The Hungry Brain" by Stephan J. Guyenet*
- *"The Body Keeps the Score" by Bessel van der Kolk*
- *"The Circadian Code" by Satchin Panda, Ph.D.*
- *"The Telomere Effect" by Elizabeth Blackburn and Elissa Epel*
- *"The Mindful Diet" by Ruth Wolever and Beth Reardon*
- *"The Microbiome Diet" by Raphael Kellman, M.D.*
- *"The Metabolism Plan" by Lyn-Genet Recitas*
- *"The Good Gut" by Justin Sonnenburg and Erica Sonnenburg*

ABOUT THE AUTHOR

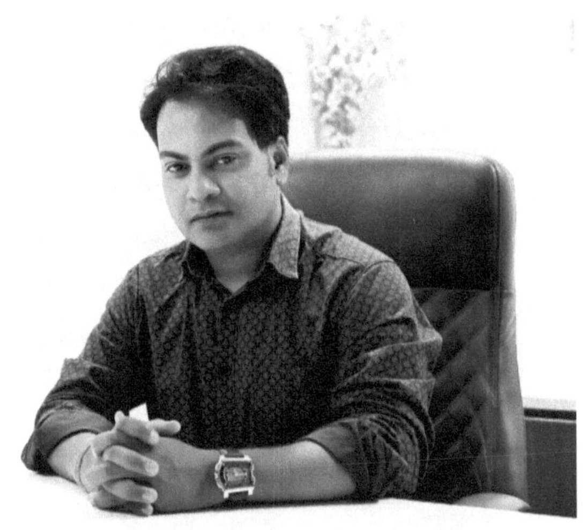

Remy Vishwakarma, the author of "Wild, Food, and Fitness: Revitalizing Modern Health with Ancestral Wisdom," is a remarkable individual whose journey from the world of Computer Application to the realm of Fitness is a testament to the power of passion and personal transformation.

Initially armed with a degree in Computer Application, Remy charted a different course when he followed his heart's true calling - Fitness. His story is one of profound personal change. At one point in his life, he grappled with a weight that exceeded 130 kilograms, confronting the physical and emotional challenges that often accompany such a burden.

However, Remy's innate curiosity and unyielding determination led him on a remarkable journey of self-discovery. He embarked on extensive research and explorations into the realms of nutrition, physical fitness, and holistic wellbeing. This voyage not only transformed his physical appearance but also revitalized his mental and emotional health.

Today, Remy stands as a living embodiment of the principles he espouses in his book. His personal journey from struggle to triumph serves as an inspirational beacon for those seeking to improve their health and wellbeing. As a co-founder of Kiran Fitness Studio (KFS), he continues to share his wisdom and passion, guiding others towards a healthier and more fulfilling life. Through "Wild, Food, and Fitness," Remy invites readers to embrace ancestral wisdom as a powerful tool to rejuvenate their modern health and embark on their unique path to holistic wellbeing.

Notes

Notes

Notes

Notes

www.ingramcontent.com/pod-product-compliance
Lightning Source LLC
Chambersburg PA
CBHW051249250726
48656CB00004B/1200